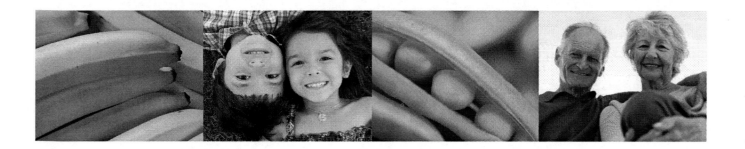

Doctors Vitamin Cures That Work

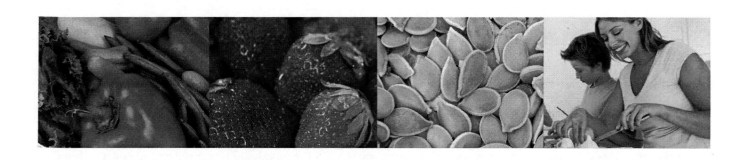

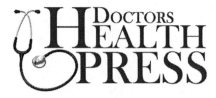

Doctors Vitamin Cures That Work
ISBN# 0-9734125-8-5

This book should not be considered a substitute for medical care from your doctor or other health care provider. This book is presented for information purposes only and should not be construed as medical advice or instruction. Please consult your doctor before undertaking any health–related activity. On any matter relating to your health or well–being, please check with an appropriate health professional. The information contained herein, while believed to be correct, is not guaranteed to be accurate or complete. Doctors Health Press and its employees are not responsible for medically unsupervised activities that could be harmful to your health.

TABLE OF
CONTENTS

Welcome...1

The State of Your Health Care 2

What Does it Cost Me? 2

What Kind of Care Am I Getting? 2

Am I the One in Control of My Health Care?........... 2

The Concept of Nationalized Health Care .. 3

An Ounce of Prevention 3

Prevention and Maintenance Are the Only
True Ways to Avoid a Crisis.............................. 3

Vitamin Therapy: The Most
Effective Choice You Can Make 4

If Vitamins Are So Great, Why Does the
Government Seem to Hate Them So Much? 4

It All Comes Back to Prevention 5

Just What Is a Vitamin, Anyway?........................... 6

What Are Minerals?... 7

Why Can't I Just Get the Vitamins
I Need from My Food? 8

5 Easy Steps to Change Your Health...................... 8

Rules in the Kitchen 9

Enter Supplements: Filling the Nutritional Gaps.... 10

Supplements and Safety..................................... 10

Are You Cooking Healthy?................................... 10

What's a "Recommended Dietary Allowance"?........ 11

Adequate Intake... 12

Estimated Average Requirement 12

Tolerable Upper Intake Level 12

Abbreviations for Dosages: What Do They Mean?... 14

VITAMINS:
THE WEAPONS IN OUR ARSENAL..........15

Vitamin A 15

What is a Free Radical? 16

Enter Beta-Carotene 16

Food Sources 17

Health Conditions 17

Beta-Carotene and Cancer 17

Vitamin A Dosage 18

Beta-Carotene.. 18

Possible Side Effects of Vitamin A 18

Toxic Dosages of Vitamin A 18

Symptoms of Acute Vitamin A Toxicity 18

Symptoms of Chronic Vitamin A Toxicity 19

Possible Side Effects of Beta-Carotene................... 19

Possible Interactions... 19

The Latest News 19

Vitamin B1 (Thiamin) 20

What Is It For?... 20

Thiamin and Alzheimer's.................................... 20

What Happens When You Don't
Get Enough? 21

Food Sources 22

Health Conditions 22

Vitamin B1 Dosage... 22

Possible Side Effects... 23

Possible Interactions... 23

The Latest News 23

Vitamin E 24

What Is It For?... 24

Vitamin B2 vs. Sickle-Cell 24
What Happens When You Don't Get Enough? 25
Food Sources 25
Health Conditions 26
Vitamin E Dosage 26
Possible Side Effects 26
Possible Interactions 26
The Latest News 26

Vitamin B3 (Niacin) 27

What Happens When You Don't Get Enough? 28
Food Sources 28
Health Conditions 28
Vitamin B3 Dosage 28
Possible Side Effects 29
Possible Interactions 29
Reynaud's Phenomenon 30
The Latest News 30

Vitamin B6 31

What Happens When You Don't Get Enough? 32
Food Sources 33
Health Conditions 33
Vitamin B6 Dosage 34
Possible Side Effects 34
Possible Interactions 34
The Latest News 34

Vitamin B9 (Folic Acid) 35

What Happens When You Don't Get Enough? 36
Food Sources 36
Health Conditions 37
Vitamin B9 Dosage 37
Possible Side Effects 37
Possible Interactions 37
The Latest News 38

Vitamin B12 39

What Happens When You Don't Get Enough? 40
Food Sources 40
Health Conditions 41

Vitamin B12 Dosage 41
Possible Side Effects 41
Possible Interactions 41
The Latest News 42

Vitamin C 43

What Happens When You Don't Get Enough? 45
Food Sources 45
Health Conditions 46
Vitamin C Dosage 46
Possible Side Effects 47
Possible Interactions 47
The Latest News 47

Vitamin D 48

What Is It For? 48
What Happens When You Don't Get Enough? 48
Food Sources 49
Health Conditions 49
Vitamin D Dosage 49
Possible Side Effects 50
Possible Interactions 51
The Latest News 51

Vitamin E 52

What Is It For? 52
What Happens When You Don't Get Enough? 53
Food Sources 53
Health Conditions 54
Vitamin E Dosage 54
Possible Side Effects 54
Possible Interactions 54
The Latest News 55

Vitamin K 56

What Is It For? 56
What Happens When You Don't Get Enough? 57
Food Sources 57
Health Conditions 58
Vitamin K Dosage 58
Possible Side Effects 58

Possible Interactions *58*
The Latest News *59*

THE MINERALS 61
Calcium 61
What Happens When You Don't Get Enough? 62
Food Sources 62
Health Conditions 62
Calcium Dosage 63
Possible Side Effects 63
Possible Interactions 64
The Latest News 64

Chromium 65
What Happens When You Don't Get Enough? 66
Food Sources 66
Health Conditions 66
Chromium Dosage 66
Possible Side Effects 67
Warnings About Interactions 67
The Latest News 67

Copper 68
What Is It For? 68
What Happens When You Don't Get Enough? 68
Food Sources 68
Health Conditions 69
Copper Dosage 69
Possible Side Effects 69
Warnings About Interactions 70
The Latest News 70

Iodine 71
What Is It For? 71
What Happens When You Don't Get Enough? 71
Food Sources 72
Health Conditions 72
Iodine Dosage 72
Possible Side Effects 73

Warnings About Interactions 73
The Latest News 74

Iron 75
What Is It For? 75
What Happens When You Don't Get Enough? 75
Food Sources 76
Health Conditions 77
Iron Dosage 77
Possible Side Effects 77
Possible Interactions 78
The Latest News 79

Magnesium 80
What Is It For? 80
What Happens When You Don't Get Enough? 81
Food Sources 81
Health Conditions 82
Magnesium Dosage 82
Possible Side Effects 83
Possible Interactions 83
The Latest News 83

Manganese 84

What Is It For? 84
What Happens When You Don't Get Enough? 84
Food Sources 85
Health Conditions 85
Manganese Dosage 86
Possible Side Effects 86
Possible Interactions 86
The Latest News 86

Potassium 87
What Is It For? 87
What Happens When You Don't Get Enough? 87
Food Sources 88
Health Conditions 88
Potassium Dosage 88
Possible Side Effects 88

Possible Interactions 89
The Latest News 89

Selenium 90

What Is It For? 90
What Happens When You Don't Get Enough? 90
Food Sources 91
Health Conditions 91
Selenium Dosage 91
Possible Side Effects 92
Possible Interactions 92
The Latest News 92

Zinc 93

What Is It For? 93
What Happens When You Don't Get Enough? 94
Food Sources 95
Health Conditions 95
Zinc Dosage 96
Possible Side Effects 96
Possible Interactions 97
The Latest News 97

THE REST OF YOUR ARSENAL: NATURAL SUPPLEMENTS, AMINO ACIDS, AND ENZYMES 99

Carnitine 99

What Is It For? 99
What Happens When You Don't Get Enough? 100
Food Sources 100
Health Conditions 101
Carnitine Dosage 101
Possible Interactions 101
The Latest News 102

Coenzyme Q10 103

What Is It For? 103
What Happens When You Don't Get Enough? 103
Food Sources 104

Health Conditions 104
Coenzyme Q10 Dosage 104
Possible Side Effects 104
Possible Interactions 105
The Latest News 105

Glucosamine 106

What Is It For? 106
What Happens When You Don't Get Enough? 106
Food Sources 106
Health Conditions 106
Glucosamine Dosage 107
Possible Side Effects 107
Possible Interactions 107
The Latest News 107

Lysine 108

What Happens When You Don't Get Enough? 108
Food Sources 108
Health Conditions 109
Lysine Dosage 109
Possible Side Effects 109
Possible Interactions 109

Proteolytic Enzymes 110

What Is It For? 110
What Happens When You Don't Get Enough? 111
Food Sources 111
Proteolytic Enzyme Dosage 111
Possible Side Effects 112
Possible Interactions 112
The Latest News 112

Quercetin 113

What Is It For? 113
What Happens When You Don't Get Enough? 113
Food Sources 113
Health Conditions 114
Quercetin Dosage 114
Possible Side Effects 114
The Latest News 114

Taurine **115**

What Is It For? 115

What Happens When You Don't Get Enough? 115

Food Sources 115

Health Conditions 116

Taurine Dosage 116

Possible Side Effects 116

Possible Interactions 116

The Latest News 116

THE BIG LIST: DEFINITIVE CURES FOR 30 CONDITIONS 117

Age Spots **117**

The Condition 117

The Causes 117

The Cure 117

Vitamins vs. Drugs and Other Treatments: A Cost Comparison 118

Alzheimer's Disease or Dementia **118**

The Condition 118

The Causes 118

The Cure 119

Vitamins vs. Drugs and Other Treatments: A Cost Comparison 119

Arteriosclerosis or Atherosclerosis **120**

The Condition 120

The Causes 120

The Cure 121

Vitamins vs. Drugs and Other Treatments: A Cost Comparison 121

Arthritis **122**

The Condition 122

The Causes 122

The Cure 122

Vitamins vs. Drugs and Other Treatments: A Cost Comparison 124

Asthma **124**

The Condition 124

The Causes 125

The Cure 125

Vitamins vs. Drugs and Other Treatments: A Cost Comparison 126

Breast Cancer **126**

The Condition 126

The Causes 126

The Cure 127

Vitamins vs. Drugs and Other Treatments: A Cost Comparison 128

Cataracts **129**

The Condition 129

The Causes 129

The Cure 129

Vitamins vs. Drugs and Other Treatments: A Cost Comparison 130

Chronic Fatigue Syndrome **131**

The Condition 131

The Causes 131

The Cure 131

Vitamins vs. Drugs and Other Treatments: A Cost Comparison 132

Chronic Obstructive Pulmonary Disease **132**

The Condition 132

The Causes 133

The Cure 133

Vitamins vs. Drugs and Other Treatments: A Cost Comparison 134

Cold Sores **134**

The Condition 134

The Cause 134

The Cure 135

Vitamins vs. Drugs and Other Treatments: A Cost Comparison 135

Congestive Heart Failure **136**

The Condition *136*
The Cause *136*
The Cure *136*
Vitamins vs. Drugs and Other Treatments:
A Cost Comparison *138*

Depression **138**

The Condition *138*
The Cause *139*
The Cure *139*
Vitamins vs. Drugs and Other Treatments:
A Cost Comparison *140*

Diabetes **140**

The Condition *140*
The Cause *141*
The Cure *141*
Vitamins vs. Drugs and Other Treatments:
A Cost Comparison *142*

Enlarged Prostate **143**

The Condition *143*
The Cause *143*
The Cure *143*
Vitamins vs. Drugs and Other Treatments:
A Cost Comparison *144*

Erectile Dysfunction **144**

The Condition *144*
The Cause *144*
The Cure *145*
Vitamins vs. Drugs and Other Treatments:
A Cost Comparison *145*

Fibromyalgia **146**

The Condition *146*
The Cause *146*
The Cure *146*
Vitamins vs. Drugs and Other Treatments:
A Cost Comparison *147*

Hemorrhoids **147**

The Condition *147*
The Cause *147*
The Cure *148*
Vitamins vs. Drugs and Other Treatments:
A Cost Comparison *148*

High Blood Pressure **149**

The Condition *149*
The Cause *149*
The Cure *149*
Vitamins vs. Drugs and Other Treatments:
A Cost Comparison *150*

High Cholesterol **151**

The Condition *151*
The Cause *152*
The Cure *152*
Vitamins vs. Drugs and Other Treatments:
A Cost Comparison *152*

Influenza **153**

The Condition *153*
The Cause *153*
The Cure *153*
Vitamins vs. Drugs and Other Treatments:
A Cost Comparison *152*

Insomnia **154**

The Condition *154*
The Cause *155*
The Cure *155*
Vitamins vs. Drugs and Other Treatments:
A Cost Comparison *156*

Macular Degeneration **156**

The Condition *156*
The Cause *156*
The Cure *157*
Vitamins vs. Drugs and Other Treatments:
A Cost Comparison *157*

Osteoporosis 158

The Condition 158
The Cause 158
The Cure 158
Vitamins vs. Drugs and Other Treatments:
A Cost Comparison 159

Prostate Cancer 160

The Condition 160
The Cause 160
The Cure 160
Vitamins vs. Drugs and Other Treatments:
A Cost Comparison 161

Shingles 161

The Condition 161
The Cause 161
The Cure 162
Vitamins vs. Drugs and Other Treatments:
A Cost Comparison 162

Sinusitis 162

The Condition 162
The Cause 163
The Cure 163
Vitamins vs. Drugs and Other Treatments:
A Cost Comparison 163

Sore Throat 164

The Condition 164
The Cause 164
The Cure 164
Vitamins vs. Drugs and Other Treatments:
A Cost Comparison 165

Tinnitus 165

The Condition 165
The Cause 165
The Cure 166
Vitamins vs. Drugs and Other Treatments:
A Cost Comparison 166

Urinary Tract Infection 167

The Condition 167
The Cause 167
The Cure 167
Vitamins vs. Drugs and Other Treatments:
A Cost Comparison 168

Vertigo 168

The Condition 168
The Cause 168
The Cure 169
Vitamins vs. Drugs and Other Treatments:
A Cost Comparison 169

Acknowledgments 170

WELCOME
AND CONGRATULATIONS

First of all, we here at Doctors Health Press want to thank you for purchasing *Doctors Vitamin Cures That Work*. The book you're holding right now contains some of the most important research to come through our office in decades.

Doctors Vitamin Cures That Work is a resource that will garner a special place in your household. It is about so much more than vitamin therapy. It gets to the root of challenges we, as human beings, face daily—the challenges that affect not just your health, but also your quality of life.

We realize you purchased this book because you have concerns you want to address: health issues you are currently experiencing, health problems you want to prevent from becoming issues, or fear and uncertainty about the future of your health care.

This book is going to address all of those concerns in a form that is easy to read, easy to reference, and easy to understand. We're going to keep the doctor-speak to a minimum, so the information is more digestible—because the better you understand how these therapies work, the more confident you will be in using them. Rest assured that the information provided in this book is a result of 20 years of research by our team of doctors.

Instead of just giving you a how-to manual, we're going to delve into a few arenas to paint a clearer picture of why this book is an important resource.

But more than anything, we want to give you the tools you need to prevent health problems, not just treat symptoms once they arise—and vitamin therapy plays a key role in doing so.

Have you ever thought about what vitamins actually are? We'll discuss that in a brief history, along with their different qualities.

We'll give you the plain talk about how vitamin therapy has been all but banned by powerful agencies and companies, and why— it's important for you to know why the cures in this book are not on everybody's lips.

By the end of this book, you will know how vitamin therapy can affect your health costs, your quality of health care, and the control of your health care, but best of all, this book will show you how vitamin therapy affects *you*, the individual.

We'll give you a rundown on each vitamin used; all the facts about them, from dosages to deficiencies; and we'll even show you where they are found naturally.

Finally, we will present the vitamin cures for 30 different diseases and conditions, how to implement them, and how to confidently include them in your daily regimen.

So on behalf of all of us here at Doctors Health Press, welcome, and thanks again.

Here's to your good health!

David Juan, M.D.

THE STATE OF YOUR HEALTH CARE

The state of your health care today is, well, not healthy! At least not as healthy as it could be. Most people have three specific worries about their health care:

1. What does it COST me?
2. What kind of CARE am I getting?
3. Am I the one in CONTROL of my health care?

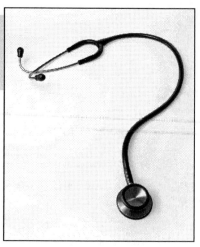

When it comes to COST, you worry about:
- How much is my co-pay?
- How much is my insurance deductible?
- What is my insurance premium?
- Does my employer provide health benefits?
- Can I afford to insure my family?
- What is the cost of my prescriptions?
- If I end up in the hospital, will it bankrupt me?
- Is it affordable to get treatment for my health issue?
- Can I afford that test, treatment, procedure, or surgery?
- Can I afford to be sick?

When it comes to CARE, you worry about:
- Will I be able to continue seeing my present doctor?
- Will I ever need to see a specialist?
- Am I always getting the utmost care from my doctor?
- Am I getting the treatments I need?
- Will the drugs I take have side effects?
- Are the drugs I'm on safe for me?
- Will I ever be able to get off prescription drugs?
- Are my prescriptions curing me, or just alleviating my symptoms?
- Do I really need that test or surgery?
- Why do I continually see my doctor, but never seem to get better?
- Does this system really want to see me well?

When it comes to CONTROL, you worry about:
- Am I in control of my care or is my doctor?
- Am I being denied care because insurance doesn't want to pay?
- Am I being denied care because a hospital is trying to cut costs?
- Is my doctor pushing drugs on me because of pharma companies?
- Does my doctor deny me care because of fear of lawsuits?
- Am I in control of my care even if I'm poor?
- Will I be in control in the future or will politicians?
- Will I be in control in the future or will insurance companies?
- Will I be in control in the future or will state exchanges?
- Will I be in control in the future or will hospitals?
- Do I have any say at all or control over my health care?

These are just some of the concerns we all share, and they can cause a lot of worry. Today these matters have become more and more confusing and muddied as more entities get involved. But above all, one thing we believe that describes the health care system like no other is prevention. Instead of looking to treat the root causes of a disease, and prevent it from developing in the first place, the industry instead just prescribes medication after medication, causing even more problems to begin with. So what can you do? It's time to practice *preventative* health care. It doesn't require expensive medications, surgeries, or intruding tests. It just requires simple changes to your lifestyle, such as making sure you're getting the right vitamins and minerals from your food and supplements to keep your brain healthy, your bones strong, and your body working well.

THE CONCEPT OF NATIONALIZED HEALTH CARE

An Ounce of Prevention...

Benjamin Franklin once said "An ounce of prevention is worth a pound of cure."

This oft-used quote extols the virtue of prevention: a little prevention now is better than having to cure something after it has already become a huge problem. This would be especially true with a disease like cancer, wouldn't it?

We do all sorts of things to fend off or prevent disease that you may not even consider preventative treatments, like bundling up for cold or rainy weather. You're trying to prevent flu, pneumonia, even the common cold. Another example is hand-sanitizing liquids. You see them on the desk of co-workers, in purses, in medicine cabinets. You use them because you are trying to prevent the transmission of germs that cause disease. You are practicing prevention.

Let's add one more term onto prevention: maintenance. We all want to maintain good health, or maintain a healthy immune system, strong bones, heart, etc. Maintenance goes hand-in-hand with prevention. We want to prevent disease, and maintain our good health.

But you may be asking, "What do prevention and maintenance have to do with the future of my health care?"

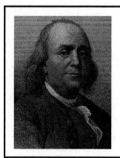

"An ounce of prevention is worth a pound of cure."
— Benjamin Franklin

Prevention and Maintenance Are the Only True Ways to Avoid a Crisis

In the 1983 movie *WarGames*, the tagline was "The only winning move is not to play."

While the tagline has been used and re-used and altered since then, its meaning is still true when dealing with an over-arching system of health care. The only way you can win is by not playing the game!

Famous comedian Henny Youngman was renowned for his huge collection of one-liners about doctors. In one of them, the patient says, "Doctor, it hurts when I do this," to which the doctor responds, "Then don't do that!"

Even though it's just a joke, the statement really sums up the whole point. If you don't want the new health care system to negatively impact your cost, care, and control of your health, then stay out of the system! To stay out of the system, simply use prevention and maintenance.

That's what this book is all about: preventing disease whenever and wherever possible, and maintaining good health. It can be done, and not by running to a doctor or emergency room every time you have the sniffles. That's not cost-effective, and frankly, it's one of the actions that have driven health care costs up so high in the first place.

You can practice prevention and maintenance in an affordable way, and that's through vitamin therapy. This book is written to explain the ins and outs of vitamin therapy and why it could be the answer you need.

Vitamin Therapy: The Most Effective Choice You Can Make

Our bodies need certain vitamins, minerals, and other substances in order to prevent disease and maintain good health. As time goes on and more scientific studies are done on vitamins, more evidence comes to light of their effectiveness for certain conditions. Continue reading for in-depth studies about the benefits of vitamins in treating 30 common conditions.

If Vitamins Are So Great, Why Does the Government Seem to Hate Them So Much?

There are numerous reasons why the government doesn't support the use of vitamins—but they aren't very good ones. This is why you hold this book in your hands right now. Let's mention some of them briefly:

Vitamins aren't drugs, so they can't be regulated

This is a big one, and for years, government offices like the Food & Drug Administration (FDA) and the American Medical Association (AMA) have been trying to amend this. Since vitamins, minerals, and amino acids are naturally occurring substances, they can't be regulated like pharmaceutical drugs can. It would be like someone trying to regulate sunlight or oxygen.

The only avenues they've had available to regulate vitamins is through their quality and production methods, or pointing to the possible toxicity that some vitamins can have when used improperly. But these are weak reasons at best.

The government doesn't make money from vitamin sales

The pharmaceutical companies make billions of dollars yearly in drug sales. They are also a huge and powerful lobbying force in Washington, D.C. Many involved in the approval of drugs for sale are themselves former employees of pharmaceutical companies or have been closely associated with them. Drug companies also pour money into campaign contributions for politicians. This makes it easier for drug companies to influence government bodies like the FDA.

Drug companies claim that their drugs are better and safer for you than vitamins. They have to. You see, if you start curing and treating yourself using vitamins, you are not buying their expensive drugs. Instead, you are opting for the cost-effective, natural way to maintain your health without the chemical toxicity and hefty bills associated with prescription drugs.

And in most cases, vitamins are as effective—if not more effective—than drugs, and they are non-toxic if used according to guidelines.

Doctors aren't taught about vitamins

Alternative medicines are simply not taught in conventional medical school. Substances such as vitamin supplements, herbal remedies, and other treatments are widely considered a "step backward" in medicine by most doctors.

Recent surveys have shown that doctors rarely even ask their patients if they are taking these kinds of remedies at all. Their training is more focused on drug and surgery therapies than natural approaches. In a survey by the Drug and Therapeutics Bulletin, 71.8% of physicians believe those who put their faith in alternatives to drugs are misguided.

If you use them, you can't be controlled

Vitamins give you a level of control over your health that is neglected by huge swaths of the population. With vitamins, there is a possibility that you will not need expensive, toxic drugs to treat your condition. You may even be able to cure your condition.

This means you have a say about what you are putting into your body, how you're combating your illness, whether you will need surgery, and the list just goes on and on. And the great thing about vitamins is that you can use them in conjunction with treatments recommended by your doctor, if you so decide. Vitamin therapy expands your control, and shrinks the control of outsiders over your health care.

They can be harmful or toxic to you

This myth has been spread around for years, especially when legislation gets proposed to try to control the vitamin industry. The propaganda and scare tactics support some of the points made above. But the truth is quite different.

You can take most vitamins by the handful and still not experience side effects or harm. The same cannot be said of pharmaceutical drugs.

The rare conditions where vitamin toxicity or side effects can occur are explained in later chapters, and you'll be taught how to avoid those situations.

It All Comes Back to Prevention

Used properly, vitamins can prevent disease and maintain your health levels. Vitamin therapy also addresses our three Cs: cost, care, and control:

Cost

Imagine avoiding doctor's visits, co-pays, prescription costs, insurance deductibles, lab tests, hospital stays, even surgeries, because your body's immune system has been repaired through vitamin therapy and is now healing itself! How much money could you save every year?

Imagine paying pennies on the dollar as opposed to the high costs of prescription drugs that only treat your symptoms.

Imagine not having to beg some insurance company for financial help because you have already prevented or eliminated a disease that could have cost you thousands.

Care

Imagine taking something that has no toxicity like pharmaceuticals…imagine having little fear of severe side effects, unlike many of today's "wonder" drugs.

Imagine not having to be exposed to radiation, deadly chemicals, or being cut into with a scalpel because you used vitamin therapy to treat or even cure your disease.

Imagine looking better, feeling younger and more energetic, your body a healing dynamo that smashes disease, enabling you to live a longer, fuller, more vital life all because of vitamin therapy.

Control

Imagine you get to decide how you're going to treat your condition, you get to dictate whether you want to fill your body with chemicals or not, and you get to actually cure ailments, not just treat their symptoms because you were able to control your health care using vitamin therapy.

With this book, you get all the control over your health care: you'll be able to look up any one of 30 different ailments and their therapies, so you'll be able to treat multiple conditions at the same time!

And best of all, you get the final say over whether you will put these therapies to work for you, and whether you will enjoy their beneficial effects. You decide—not the politicians; not the AMA, the United States Department of Health and Human Services (HHS), the FDA, or other bureaucrats; not the lawyers; and not the medical establishment. You get the final word.

VITAMINS 1

Just What Is a Vitamin, Anyway?

Believe it or not, vitamins weren't discovered until the 20th century!

For thousands of years, people ate certain foods and eventually took notice of how different foods affected the body. As time progressed, they could also see how consuming various foods helped them avoid or impact disease. They knew that there was something inside the food that blocked disease; they just couldn't identify what it was.

Then in 1905, an English doctor named William Fletcher discovered that if certain factors were removed from foods, it would result in disease. Dr. Fletcher was observing those suffering from the disease called beriberi and noticed that those who ate rice that was polished contracted beriberi while those eating unpolished rice didn't. Since the only difference was having the husk of the grain intact in the case of the unpolished rice, Dr. Fletcher believed that there must have been nutrients in the husk that protected against the disease.

This theory was further explored, and Sir Frederick Gowland Hopkins, an English biochemist, identified other "food factors" in 1906.

It wasn't until 1912 that these food factors finally had a name: vitamins. A Polish scientist named Casimir Funk created the term. He formulated the word from *vita*, meaning "life," and *amine*, which was short for thiamine. Funk had discovered thiamine in the husks of rice, and was deriving compounds from the thiamine itself. So, the actual word he created was "vitamine," which was shortened to vitamin.

Hopkins and Funk both put forth the theory of deficiency—that if you are lacking in certain vitamins, you will get sick.

It is important to remember that a vitamin has two aspects:

1. It is a substance vital to human health
2. The body alone cannot synthesize a vitamin

To synthesize means to create or formulate, so our bodies don't create vitamins. Rather, vitamins are present in our food, like the rice husks that Dr. Fletcher originally studied. With time, all 13 vitamins were isolated from food sources and identified, although not all at once. The following is a list of vitamins and when they were discovered:

Vitamin A (Retinol): 1912–1914
Vitamin B1 (Thiamine): 1929
Vitamin B2 (Riboflavin): 1926
Vitamin B3 (Niacin): 1937
Vitamin B9 (Folic Acid): 1933
Vitamin B5 (Pantothenic Acid): 1933
Vitamin B6 (Pyridoxine): 1934
Vitamin B7 (Biotin): 1931
Vitamin B12 (Cobalamins): 1934
Vitamin C (Ascorbic Acid): 1912
Vitamin D (Calciferol): 1922
Vitamin E (Tocopherol): 1922

Once the chemical compositions of each of these were broken down, scientists were then able to synthesize them in a laboratory, or extract them from food, to be put into capsules. Thus, the first vitamin supplements were created. For the most part, they've remained unchanged to this day.

What Are Minerals?

Scientists in the 1930s were attempting to get to the root cause of a type of anemia that was striking a particular group: teenage girls. The condition called chlorosis was only afflicting those girls who were deficient in iron. Their red blood cells didn't have enough iron; therefore, those cells weren't carrying enough oxygen to all parts of the body, which is what our hemoglobin does. Iron is also necessary to create new blood cells.

This case brought minerals to the scientific forefront as vitamins had been years earlier. And like vitamins, minerals have critical roles in the body's health and function. We've always gotten minerals into our system through water, plants, and animals. Minerals are a part of the very earth we inhabit. Minerals in the water are taken into plants, which use the water to grow. Animals drink the water, or consume the plants, causing them to ingest minerals as well. As humans, we drink water and consume plants and animals, deriving minerals from all three sources.

Minerals differ from vitamins in some other ways—vitamins are organic, while minerals are inorganic substances. Minerals are also considered micronutrients, because your body needs much smaller quantities as opposed to vitamins.

There are two classifications of minerals: macro and micro. The macro group includes:

Calcium

Magnesium

Phosphorus

Potassium

Chloride

Sodium

Sulfur

These are powerful minerals that are found within your body in large quantities.

The *micro* minerals (also called trace minerals) are needed in smaller amounts. Examples of these would be:

Chromium

Copper

Iodine

Iron

Manganese

Selenium

Zinc

There is no difference in importance between the two groups: your body needs all of them equally. However, the major minerals are needed in quantities of 250 milligrams (mg) a day, whereas the trace elements are only needed in doses of 20 micrograms (mcg) daily.

Another group of minerals are the electrolytes. Electrolytes channel the energy that your body needs to function. Think of them as helping your body's electrical wiring. They assist your muscles in contracting, and help transmit nerve impulses. Here is a list of electrolytes:

Potassium

Sodium (salt)

Magnesium

Chloride

VITAMINS 1

Our bodies would stop working without minerals because we wouldn't form the enzymes that govern our chemical and physiological processes. We wouldn't be able to transport oxygen to our cells. The same enzymes also control the balance of acids and bases, as well as our fluid balance. Minerals like calcium are critical to our underlying bone structure, and are components of many other bodily compounds.

Why Can't I Just Get the Vitamins I Need from My Food?

There are some very stark realities that have changed the way we eat, and what is in our food. The sad reality is that many people don't even cook anymore, opting instead for easy-to-prepare processed foods, microwavable foods, or fast food. Many cite a lack of time, energy, or even the funds to eat good healthy food.

Processed food or convenience foods are devoid of nutritional value. It takes only a minute to prove this to yourself by examining the ingredients on the label of a processed food (something you are not cooking fresh or from scratch). You will see the names of chemicals. You will see dyes listed (to give the product appealing color). You will see preservatives (high sodium contents or monosodium glutamate [MSG], to give the food a longer shelf life). You will see artificial flavorings (to add taste). But, despite advertising campaigns that make these products look good and healthy for you, these products can actually harm you, because they're devoid of the vitamins and minerals that your body desperately needs.

Your body needs vitamins and minerals to run properly. Processed foods don't put the essential nutrients into your body that you would get from fresh food. Eating these convenience foods over the years has made us an obese, fatigued, unhealthy society. Our bodies

5 Easy Steps to Change Your Health

1. Eat more fruits and vegetables every day: Fruits and vegetables are packed with the fuel your body needs to keep you healthy. Whenever you eat them, keep in mind that, in general, the rawer they are, the more nutrients you get.

2. Eat fresh meats and fish: Eat meats in moderation, and change up your diet regularly to get the proper ratio of what you need, including healthy fats. Be careful when preparing meats and make sure to add fresh fish to your diet.

3. Eat whole grains, not refined grains: Processed foods use a lot of white flour, because it allows for longer shelf life. Unfortunately, the process used to make white flour effectively removes nutrients. Opting for whole grains instead will help you get the nutrients you need.

4. Eat more legumes: Legumes (beans and seeds) are packed with protein, vitamins, fiber, and essential minerals. Plus, they are cheap to buy, and are low in saturated fats, cholesterol, and calories.

5. Eat with variety: Shake up your diet whenever possible to ensure that your body is getting a steady flow of all different types of nutrients.

are starved for vitamins and minerals. Processed foods may solve a time or convenience problem in our lives, but in the long run, we'll pay dearly for it. Sadly, with many foods, we are merely putting matter into our stomachs that not only is unable to fortify our bodies, but that is confusing our bodily functions and damaging our organs by trying to get our systems to process chemicals that don't normally appear in the food chain.

To be healthy, you need to start treating your body right. Before we start talking about the vitamin cures for your everyday illnesses, here are some simple things you can do every day that take only a little effort—and will help you reap big rewards.

Rules in the Kitchen

Although there are some foods that are difficult to eat raw, you can cook them in a way to gain the optimum nutrient levels. There are some basic guidelines you can use when preparing vegetables and other items.

Vitamins dissolve more quickly in water than minerals do. When you boil food, remember that the longer you leave it in, the more vitamins and minerals will dissolve out of it. With vegetables, there can be a large loss of minerals. This is especially true if you add salt to the water. The salt leaches out calcium, potassium, and sodium. Use the least amount of water possible, and try not to boil anything longer than 20 minutes.

Blanching also causes nutrient loss. Blanching is often used to maintain color for certain vegetables by quickly boiling them, then transferring them to icy-cold water to "halt" the cooking process.

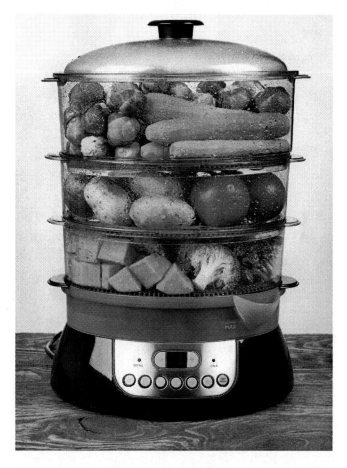

When cooking vegetables, especially root vegetables, you should try to leave the skin on, or peel it thinly. The area directly under the skin is the most nutrient-packed area of the vegetable. Remember too, that once you peel vegetables and fruit, oxidation starts to occur, so cook them right away to maximize their benefits. Air destroys nutrients just as boiling does.

The worst way to cook vegetables is by microwaving them. For instance, broccoli is one of the most nutrient-dense vegetables around. But when you microwave it, it loses 75%–90% of its nutrients. By comparison, if you were to steam the broccoli, it would lose between zero and 10% of its nutrient value.

VITAMINS 1

Steaming will give you the most beneficial results with vegetables, as it keeps the minerals locked in the food. When cooking rice, make sure you try to use the exact amount of water needed to cook the grains. This way, the rice can suck back up any vitamins or minerals that are pulled into the boiling water as it expands.

Finally, a great way to cook is with cast-iron pots and pans. While this was more common in the past than it is today, cooking with cast-iron is healthful because iron from the cookware will actually be added to the food. This is good news, since iron deficiency is a common problem in North America, especially for new and pregnant mothers.

Enter Supplements: Filling the Nutritional Gaps

In modern society, it sometimes is simply impossible to get all the vitamins, minerals, and other substances we need in order to maintain our best healthful state. In fact, eight out of 10 people in the U.S. do not get enough fruits and vegetables in their diets. That is a huge number of people whose health is being negatively impacted. This is one reason why supplements can fill your body's vital need for vitamins and minerals.

But there are even more chemicals and substances that keep the machinery of our body in working order that we can also get in supplement form, like amino acids, enzymes, and even beneficial herbs.

Supplements are a great boon to people on special diets who may be missing the nutrients they would get from their foods, such as vegetarians, vegans, or those on popular low-carb or low-fat diets.

People with certain conditions are now able to use supplements to fill the gaps in their nutritional intake. What's even better is that they are now able to put supplements to work in preventing or fighting disease.

Supplements and Safety

Although most supplements are safe, and in many cases far safer than prescription drugs, there are some guidelines to know and follow when using them:

Are You Cooking Healthy?

1. Broccoli when blanched loses 47% of its vitamin C

2. Carrots when boiled lose 80% of their folate

3. Cauliflower when boiled loses 70% of its folate

4. Mixed vegetables boiled for 10–20 minutes lose 55% of their vitamin C

5. Navy beans when cooked lose between 50% and 70% of every mineral

6. Soybeans when boiled lose up to 75% of their vitamin B1 content

7. Spinach when boiled loses 50% of its flavonoids

Read Labels Carefully

The label will instruct you on the proper and best use of the supplement. It may direct you to take it with meals, when to take it, how many to take, and so on. Before you purchase a supplement, you should have an idea of your nutritional needs. For instance, vegans don't get enough vitamin B12 through diet alone, so purchasing this supplement is probably a good idea for them.

Store Supplements Wisely

Keep them away from young children, as you would with a prescription drug. Store supplements in a cool, dry place. They should not be kept in the bathroom, due to humidity and possible steam from showering.

Don't Be Fooled by "Megadoses"

Many supplement products boast of being packed with a "megadose" of any number of vitamins and/or minerals. Anything more than 100% of your daily requirement could be counter-productive, since you will also be getting some of these substances in your diet anyway.

While many vitamins are safe even at high doses, other nutrients can be toxic in excessive amounts. Plus, your body doesn't need excessive amounts of all nutrients; your body will merely shed the extra vitamins and minerals through urination rather than putting all of them to use. Know, too, that some companies use megadoses simply to drive up the cost of their supplements.

Look for "USP"

These letters on a package mean that the supplement has been recognized by the United States Pharmacopeia (USP) agency for effectiveness, purity, and other factors.

Watch Expiration Dates

Some vitamins will have an expiration date because they lose potency over time. Avoid those that don't have one, and don't use any vitamins that have expired.

Talk to Your Doctor

If you are trying to use certain supplements to combat a medical condition, or if you believe you are suffering from a deficiency, it would be wise to discuss it with your doctor first. They can let you know if the intake of certain vitamins or minerals will have a negative impact on your condition or not. As stated earlier, vitamins and minerals can have their own side effects in different situations.

What's a "Recommended Dietary Allowance"?

Governments have tried to determine what amounts of vitamins and nutrients we need to remain healthy. This hasn't been an easy task, since we all differ in age, sex, life situations, size, shape, weight, level of health, and so on. The government has attempted to come up with standardized guidelines for the population to follow, but as of this time, they've still not perfected them.

The U.S. Food and Nutrition Board (FNB), a division of the National Academy of Sciences, undertook the first attempt to standardize guidelines in the 1940s. The FNB created the first Recommended Dietary Allowance, or (RDA). The RDA is a result of roughly calculating how much of a particular nutrient you need each day, with an added amount for assurance. The FNB then tried to tweak those amounts based on whether you are a man or woman, a child, adolescent, adult, or even a pregnant or lactating woman.

The allowances are meant to ensure that over time, you will not become deficient in that singular nutrient. RDAs do not exist for all nutrients, so it's been the position of the National Academy of Sciences that your diet should include a wide variety of foods to help ensure your body gets what it needs to remain healthy.

Adding Confusion to the Mix

In 1997, the Institute of Medicine of the National Academies (or the IOM) released a list of changes in the allowances for different nutrients. The IOM also decided to change the term "Recommended Dietary Allowance" to "Dietary Reference Intake," or DRI.

One of the main reasons the IOM gave for the change was that it wanted the term to take into consideration common medical conditions that were shared among people, besides age and sex.

DRIs have not been formulated for all nutrients yet. It's important to note the new categories that resulted from the IOM's report, and what these new recommendations mean when we are looking at DRIs:

Adequate Intake

This category is meant to cover you when a proper RDA hasn't been scientifically determined for a nutrient. It tells you how much

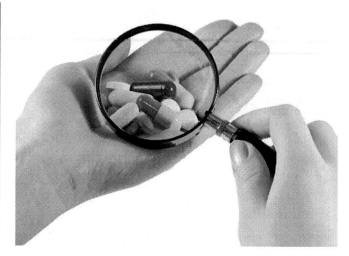

of that nutrient will assist you in maintaining good health, even when a definite allowance hasn't been calculated. In these cases, science simply does not yet know enough about the nutrient to set up allowances.

Estimated Average Requirement

This estimate is for a level that will maintain half the individuals in a group based on sex or age. Think of this number as having a 50% accuracy rate.

Tolerable Upper Intake Level

This is the ceiling or maximum dosage level for each age and sex group. Anything exceeding this suggested level could start to cause health problems.

These three new recommendations sprang from the additional research the IOM did after RDAs were first calculated. To demonstrate the difference between the two standards, let's compare the two charts side by side. Here are RDA and DRI charts for calcium:

Calcium

RDA*

Infants (0–1 year)	500 mg
Children (1–10 y)	800 mg
Males (11–24 y)	1,200 mg
Males (25–51+ y)	800 mg
Females (11–24 y)	1,200 mg
Females (25–51+ y)	800 mg
Pregnant Females	1,200 mg
Breastfeeding Mothers	1,200 mg

DRI**

Infants (0–6 months)	210 mg
Infants (7–12 mo.)	270 mg
Children (1–3 y)	500 mg
Children (4–8 y)	800 mg
Males (9–18 y)	1,300 mg
Males (19–50 y)	1,000 mg
Males (51+)	1,200 mg
Females (9–18 y)	1,300 mg
Females (19-50 y)	1,000 mg
Females (51+)	1,200 mg
Pregnant Females (under 18 y)	1,300 mg
Pregnant Females (19–50 y)	1,000 mg
Breastfeeding Mothers (under 18 y)	1,300 mg
Breastfeeding Mothers (19–50 y)	1,000 mg

* The RDA chart changes between vitamins and minerals, sometimes simply saying men/women over the age of 18, or even over the age of 12, rather than splitting up fewer than 24 and over 25 as the calcium RDA example does above.

** All have an Upper Intake level set at 2,500 mg a day.

Additional notes that appear on the above example DRI for calcium:

Function: Essential in blood clotting, muscle contraction, nerve transmission, and bone and teeth formation

Adverse Effects of Excess Calcium: Kidney stones, hypercalcemia, milk alkali syndrome, renal insufficiency

Special Consideration: Amenorrheic women have reduced calcium absorption; no consistent data to support that a high protein intake increases calcium requirement.

There are those who believe that both sets of recommendations are still too low, and are not ensuring that people are getting enough of their daily intake of vitamins and minerals.

If you are trying to maintain optimum health, and if you are trying to prevent disease before it occurs, you may want to consider RDAs and DRIs on the low end and act accordingly. There are many vitamins and minerals that are so beneficial to your immune system, like antioxidants, that you simply cannot get too much of them.

Toxicity for vitamins and minerals is usually much higher than you could ever achieve, and for those substances that pose any kind of toxicity risk, we've carefully mentioned them in our rundown of the different vitamins and minerals further on in this book.

Besides, very few people can possibly go about their daily activity and be able to calculate their daily allowances for all the different nutrients. If you eat well and really listen to what your body is telling you, you should never have to be overly concerned about tracking your daily allowances.

Abbreviations for Dosages: What Do They Mean?

In this book, you will see recommended dosages for supplementing with vitamins and minerals. At first glance, they can look kind of confusing. So let's take a quick look at the ones you'll see here, and what they mean. You'll see these on the labels, and most are very specific depending on the substance:

Milligrams (mg)

One milligram (mg) is a thousandth, or 1/1000, of a gram (g). So when you see "mg," think "smaller than a gram," or 1 mg < 1 g.

Micrograms (mcg)

This dosage is smaller yet. One microgram (mcg) is equal to one-thousandth, or 1/1000, of a milligram. It is also one millionth of a gram—quite a tiny dosage indeed. When you see the "mcg" measurement, you can think "smaller than a milligram," or 1 mcg < 1 mg.

International Units (IU)

This one tends to be very confusing. Unlike mg and mcg, which are portions of a gram, international units (IU) are units that are used to measure *potency*, not *quantity*. They are specific to certain substances due to their activity in your body, not their weight or volume. For instance, vitamins A and D are usually expressed in IU.

As opposed to mg or mcg, an IU does not convert readily into set measurements. For instance, while we know 1,000 x 1 mg = 1 g,

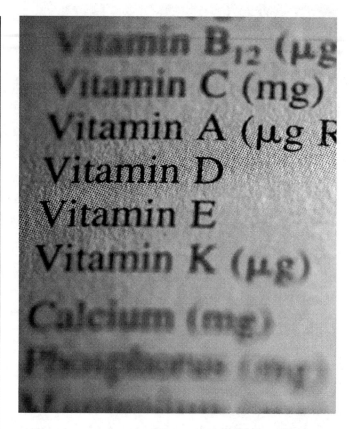

one IU can equal 0.3 mcg of retinol, 0.6 mcg of beta-carotene, or 1.2 mcg of other provitamin-A carotenoids. In simple terms, one IU of vitamin D does not equal one IU of vitamin E.

International units were created to express a value for the effect that different substances have on the body; in other words, the acting property from one IU of a substance equals the same effect on the body as one IU of another. If it still sounds confusing, don't worry, just stick to the recommended dosage on the label. If you have any questions about taking more than the recommended dosage, consult your doctor.

VITAMINS:
THE WEAPONS IN OUR ARSENAL

Vitamin A

What Is It For?

Besides being essential for your body in general, let's focus on the specific benefits of vitamin A:

Immune System Support

The first line of defense for your body's immune system includes your skin, the mucous membranes in your nose and throat, and tissues in your gastrointestinal organs. These serve to block germs, viruses, and other bacteria before they can take hold and make you sick.

Vitamin A strengthens that first line of defense. That's why using this vitamin can actually help you avoid colds and other viral infections. Vitamin A is also an antioxidant, a molecule that prevents the oxidation of other molecules. The oxidation of tissue in our bodies is normal, but damaging to our cells, which is why we need antioxidants like vitamin A for our immune system to be effective. Vitamin A is known to combat free radicals (see sidebar on the next page).

Cell Reproduction

Vitamin A helps cells reproduce. The scientific name for cell reproduction is "differentiation." If a cell doesn't go through differentiation, it can mutate or change in a negative way. These cells can mutate into cancer cells. So in addition to protecting your cells from free radicals, vitamin A can also help them reproduce normally.

Our reproductive functions are also supported by vitamin A. The vitamin helps the ovaries and formulation of placenta in women, and promotes a man's sperm creation.

Good Eyesight

Our eyes take in light and transmit it into signals that run from our optic nerve to the brain. Our brain then interprets the signals as visual pictures, enabling us to see what is around us, the colors of our surrounding, whether there is lots of light or if it's dark, and so on.

The retinas of our eyes are fortified by a supply of vitamin A that gathers in the retina. The vitamin ensures that the retina is functioning properly, especially when it adjusts from environments of bright light to darkness. Night blindness can occur when the retina is damaged.

Dry eyes can also be treated with vitamin A eye drops.

Healthy Skin

Vitamin A doesn't just help your skin on the inside by boosting your immune system; it can also keep your skin stay healthy on the outside as well. Your skin is the largest organ of your body, and you can heal cuts, scrapes, burns, and even cold sores by applying vitamin A topically (putting it in direct contact with the skin) in the form of a cream or lotion.

Blood Sugar

Even people who eat the right foods can still have blood sugar (blood-glucose) problems. A trial study of elderly people with type 2 diabetes showed a significant lack of vitamin A—even with a proper diet.[1] Supplementing with vitamin A can solve this problem.

Enter Beta-Carotene

Although most vitamins are safely taken without fear of overdosing, care must be taken with vitamin A, because it can be toxic in large amounts. This is because vitamin A is fat-soluble, whereas others are water-soluble. Water-soluble vitamins are expelled with your urine when they are present in an excess amount. Since vitamin A is stored in fat, it remains in your body.

However, you can avoid this problem by upping your intake of beta-carotene. Beta-carotene can be found in many food sources and in supplement (pill) form as well. Beta-carotene is known as a provitamin, because it is not actually vitamin A, but your body converts it into vitamin A. Beta-carotene is also a water-soluble nutrient, so there is little fear of toxicity.

The molecules of beta-carotene are similar to vitamin A. When your body is low in vitamin A, an enzyme in your intestines breaks the beta-carotene molecules in half, resulting in two molecules of vitamin A.

Beta-carotene was discovered by scientists who were curious about the properties of colorful plants in nature. It was synthesized, and then sold as a supplement in the 1950s, even before all of its beneficial properties were known.

What Is a Free Radical?

Free radicals are chemically active fragments of molecules. They have a different electrical charge than other molecules in your body, because they have either too many electrons or too few.

Free radicals damage your other cells by stealing their electrons or adding excess electrons to them. The effect damages your cells, protein, and DNA. The damage is called "oxidation." It's the process you see when a sliced apple turns brown or a piece of iron rusts.

Our bodies can form free radicals naturally, through our respiration, metabolism, or tissue inflammation. We can also take in free radicals from outside the body through sunlight, smoking, alcohol, strenuous exercise, x-rays, and pollution.

Normally, a healthy immune system can counteract free radicals, but since oxidation has a cumulative effect over time, we are susceptible to more damage as we age. Boosting our immune systems with antioxidants can help.

It's believed antioxidants combat chronic diseases, such as cancer, heart disease, stroke, Alzheimer's, rheumatoid arthritis, and cataracts.

Food Sources

Here are the foods we can derive vitamin A from:

- Cheese
- Butter
- Fortified (vitamin A added) margarine
- Cream
- Fortified milk
- Fortified breakfast cereals
- Liver
- Cod liver oil
- Egg yolks

Note: In the case of "fortified" foods, the label may list the vitamin A source as "retinol."

Here are foods that contain beta-carotene:

- Broccoli
- Dark green leafy vegetables: spinach, kale, collard greens, cilantro, turnip greens
- Orange and yellow vegetables: carrots, winter squash, sweet potatoes, bell peppers
- Orange and yellow fruits: cantaloupe, apricots, oranges

Health Conditions

Vitamin A is useful in treating these various conditions:

- Poor eyesight, night blindness
- Weakened immune system
- Cold, flu, and other viral infections
- Cancer
- Diabetes
- Reproductive health
- Cuts, scrapes, and cold sores

Beta-carotene is beneficial for these conditions:

- Weakened immune system
- Heart disease
- Arterial plaque
- Cancer
- Cataracts, macular degeneration
- Osteoarthritis, rheumatoid arthritis
- Depression
- Asthma
- Headaches
- Cystic fibrosis
- Heartburn
- Infertility
- Psoriasis
- Epilepsy
- Sunburn

Beta-Carotene and Cancer

This section is of special note since there is a lot of contradictory

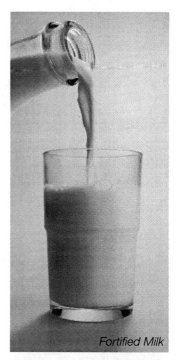

Fortified Milk

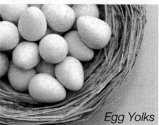

Egg Yolks

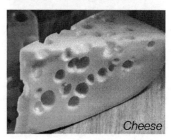

Cheese

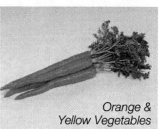

Orange & Yellow Vegetables

VITAMINS 1

information about beta-carotene's abilities as a cancer preventive. In supplement form, some studies have concluded that there is no link between beta-carotene and cancer prevention.

There have even been studies concluding that beta-carotene can actually increase the risk of cancer in certain groups of people, mainly smokers and those who consume high amounts of alcohol. A study from Finland of 30,000 male smokers found that supplementing with beta-carotene increased their risk of lung cancer by almost 20%.[2]

Still, others tout the anti-cancer effects of beta-carotene in different groups, especially those eating raw vegetables. This may be due to the fact that other carotenoids in these fruits and vegetables may work in conjunction with beta-carotene to slam cancer cells. "Mixed" supplements are now available that can mimic the effects of the natural equivalent.

At the very least, we know that the vitamin A that beta-carotene produces is an antioxidant, one that promotes healthy cells and fights the free radicals that have been tied to cancer.

Dosage

Vitamin A

Recommended Daily Intake (Men):	1,000 mg
Recommended Daily Intake (Women):	800 mg
Daily Intake (Pregnant Women):	Not Recommended
Maximum Recommended Intake:	5,000 mg or lower

Beta-Carotene

There is no current hard information about recommended intake levels, although most supplements contain 15 mg per day. However, you can feel free to get your beta-carotene by eating the right vegetables and fruit.

Possible Side Effects of Vitamin A

Since vitamin A is a fat-soluble vitamin as opposed to beta-carotene, it's important to be cautious about overdosing, causing toxicity in your system. The medical term for this is *hypervitaminosis A*. This happens when you take too many vitamin A supplements or eat too many vitamin A-rich foods like liver.

Toxic Dosages of Vitamin A

Children:	25,000 IU
Adults:	50,000 IU

Toxicity is classified as being either acute or chronic. Acute toxicity describes a short-term problem where you have taken in an excessive amount of vitamin A and your body is feeling effects within a few hours or days. Chronic toxicity describes long-term effects similar to what one could expect from taking continually high doses of vitamin A over months and years. These dosages would be much higher, more along the lines of 100,000 IU or 30,000 mg regularly. Chronic toxicity is much more dangerous than acute toxicity.

Symptoms of Acute Vitamin A Toxicity

- Dizziness
- Vomiting

- Blurred vision
- Muscle pain
- Fatigue
- Nausea
- Irritability
- Headache
- Abdominal pain
- Lack of concentration, hard to think

Symptoms of Chronic Vitamin A Toxicity

- Bone pain/swelling
- Hair loss
- Liver damage
- Irritability
- Insomnia
- Headache
- Weight loss
- Loss of appetite/anorexia
- High cholesterol
- Vision problems
- Fatigue
- Fever
- Anemia
- Skin dryness/itchiness
- Increased risk of osteoporosis

Possible Side Effects of Beta-Carotene

As we've mentioned a little earlier, some researchers theorize that beta-carotene can actually increase free radicals in certain individuals. However, there is no definitive information at this time.

The only known side effects of getting too much beta-carotene are:

- Diarrhea
- Yellowish color on hands and feet

This would occur if you were supplementing at an amount of 20 mg or more daily. If you are getting your beta-carotene through diet, you don't have to worry about side effects at all.

Possible Interactions

Don't take supplements of vitamin A or beta-carotene if you:

- Smoke
- Take the acne drug "Accutane" (an extremely high dose of vitamin A)
- Are pregnant
- Take anticonvulsants
- Take "Warfarin"
- Take retinoids
- Take tetracycline antibiotics

Due to possible toxicity concerns with vitamin A supplements and a lack of study information on supplemental beta-carotene, you should consult your doctor before adding these to your vitamin regimen.

The Latest News

In a 2011 study conducted by researchers at the Fox Chase Cancer Center, a possible key to fighting breast cancer in its early stages was found in retinoic acid, a derivative of vitamin A. Further studies are ongoing, but it appears to suppress tumors, even reversing the growth of abnormal masses in the breast.

VITAMINS 1

Vitamin B1 (Thiamin)

What Is It For?

Your body needs thiamin in order to process carbohydrates, proteins, and fats. Here are some of thiamin's other functions:

Energy and Metabolism

When you eat, your body breaks the food down into the components it needs, including energy. Some of this energy will be used to meet immediate needs, and some will be stored in the body for later use. The carbohydrates, proteins, and fats from your food raise your blood sugar, but it needs to be converted into energy.

Your cells can't carry the energy you need unless they have a molecule called ATP (adenosine triphosphate). This is where vitamin B1 comes in. The vitamin B1 in your system enables your cells to create the ATP molecules they need to convert blood sugar into energy and carry it throughout your body. Vitamin B1 also kickstarts your body's enzymes that break down carbohydrates.

Brain Function

Your brain uses glucose to function properly. Since thiamin converts glucose (blood sugar) into energy, it's not hard to assume that a lack of vitamin B1 in your system could impair your normal brain function. Thiamin can clear up that "fuzzy thinking."

The brain uses chemicals called neurotransmitters to carry signals to and from your body. These chemicals may also depend on thiamin for proper formation. A neurotransmitter called acetylcholine is needed for memory and mental performance.

Animal studies have shown that a deficiency in vitamin B1 leads to lack of memory and response to stimuli. This may describe a human disease called beriberi. Sufferers find themselves weak, fatigued, and unmotivated, with difficulty in forming thoughts and a general disinterest in what's going on around them. Beriberi is an East Asian word meaning, "I can't, I can't."

Heart Health

When the heart doesn't pump blood the way it should, over time you can develop congestive heart failure. The name doesn't mean that your heart has stopped; just that it's not moving blood to parts of your body the way it should. For instance, if the right side of your heart is not pumping properly, you won't get enough blood to your lungs. If the left side is impaired, the

---

Thiamin and Alzheimer's

Alzheimer's disease degenerates your nerve receptors, also called the cholinergic system.

Since vitamin B1 also affects this system, continual studies are being done to determine if thiamin can have a positive impact on Alzheimer's sufferers.

Although no conclusive link has been found between the two, we can hope that thiamin will one day play a vital role in stopping the spread of this cruel and incurable disease.

---

rest of your body suffers from a lack of blood. Heart failure can involve both sides.

Thiamin has a definite positive impact on your heart. In one double-blind study, 30 people who had suffered congestive heart failure were given intravenous (IV) doses of vitamin B1. Those who took in 200 mg a day experienced improved cardiac health.[3]

What Happens When You Don't Get Enough?

When you are mildly deficient in vitamin B1, you may experience the following symptoms:

- Mood swings
- Feelings of fear, anxiety
- Depression
- Confusion
- Loss of appetite
- Insomnia
- Muscle weakness
- Weight loss
- Abdominal pain
- Loss of memory

In cases of severe vitamin B1 deficiency, you may have these symptoms:

- Nerve pain
- Paralysis
- Swelling of the hands and legs
- Difficulty breathing

If you have an impaired ability to absorb thiamin, you may contract the disease beriberi. Beriberi is uncommon today compared to the past, but it hasn't been eradicated entirely. Beriberi is broken into two categories, each with its own set of symptoms. One form is called dry and the other wet.

Dry Beriberi

This category indicates developing muscle and nerve problems. It affects the large muscle groups in your legs, so you may notice general pain and weakness there. You may also feel a "pins and needles" sensation in your toes, and/or a burning sensation in your feet.

Wet Beriberi

This category is more dangerous, since it can cause problems for your heart. Symptoms include dilation of the blood vessels, a feeling of warmth and moistness in the skin, false heart rates, and an over-pumping of blood by the heart. Continual overworking of your heart will lead to congestive heart failure accompanied by congestion in your lungs and edema (swelling) in your legs. This will also play havoc with your blood pressure, resulting in spikes and drops.

Alcohol and Thiamin

Alcohol abuse increases the risk of thiamin deficiency. This happens on two levels. Alcoholics have notoriously bad diets, either ignoring food altogether or lacking vitamin B1 in the foods they do eat. Also, alcohol causes vitamin B1 to be excreted quickly, depleting the body's stores of this nutrient. An alcohol binge can cause such a huge drop in thiamin levels that it results in brain abnormalities. The danger exists in sudden surges of thiamin levels as well. For instance, an alcoholic who suddenly wakes up in the hospital may find themselves being fed with an IV. This could cause a spike in their body's thiamin levels.

Food Sources

Here are the foods we can derive vitamin B1 from:

- Yeasts (baker's and brewer's)
- Whole grain breads
- Asparagus
- Enriched flour
- Crimini mushrooms
- Legumes (navy beans, pinto beans, kidney beans, and peas)
- Lean pork, ham, and liver
- Wheat germ
- Nuts (peanuts are an especially good source)
- Fish (tuna is an excellent source)
- Brussels sprouts
- Romaine lettuce

Health Conditions

Vitamin B1 is useful in treating the following conditions:

- Low energy
- Low metabolism
- Memory loss
- Low brain function, confusion
- Alzheimer's disease
- Nerve function
- Congestive heart failure
- Mood swings
- Anxiety
- Depression
- Insomnia
- Muscle weakness
- Weight loss
- Abdominal pain
- Edema of hands, feet, and legs
- Blood vessel dilation
- False heart rate
- Swings in blood pressure

Dosage

Vitamin B1, Thiamin Hydrochloride, Thiamin Nitrate

Recommended Daily Intake (Men):	1.5 mg
Recommended Daily Intake (Women):	1.1 mg
Recommended Intake:	200 mg

Some supplements may contain as much as 5 mg daily. This is absolutely fine, since there is nothing to show that vitamin B1 causes toxicity of any kind, nor has an official maximum dose been established. Likewise, pregnant women and children can take it without fear.

Possible Side Effects

Any concern about vitamin B1 is related to intravenous (IV) doses. There have been occasional reports of serious reactions, but these are probably due to allergic reactions from patients. An allergic reaction can result in anaphylactic shock.

However, this book deals with supplements in pill form. And in the case of thiamin, or vitamin B1, users have nothing to be concerned about.

Possible Interactions

There are no known interactions with vitamin B1.

The Latest News

A recent study of college-aged women showed that they had improved moods, energy, and alertness after taking doses of thiamin at 50 mg daily for two months. Although the women weren't thiamin deficient, they still experienced benefits that seem to point to effectiveness in using thiamin to treat depression.

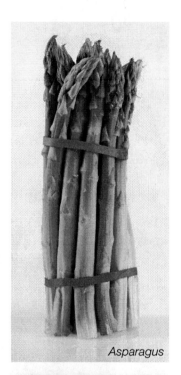

Asparagus

Wernicke-Korsakoff Syndrome

Thiamin deficiency in alcoholics can result in Wernicke-Korsakoff syndrome, a brain disorder. The syndrome damages the central nervous system. Those afflicted may engage in confabulation (making up falsehoods to explain erratic behavior) with no memory of even doing so. Here are some other symptoms:

- Drooping eyelids
- Unsteady walking
- Double vision
- Hallucinations
- Loss of muscle coordination

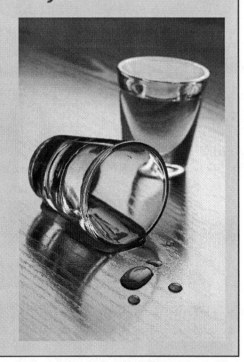

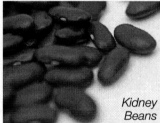

Kidney Beans

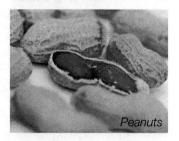

Peanuts

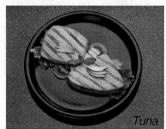

Tuna

VITAMINS 1

Vitamin E

What Is It For?

Vitamin B2 is an essential vitamin that helps with energy, metabolism, cellular support, and many chemical reactions in your body.

Energy and Metabolism

Like its cousin B1, vitamin B2 also helps your body convert carbohydrates, proteins, and fats into ATP, the energy molecule your cells need.

Cellular Support

In addition to processing fats and amino acids, vitamin B2 is needed to create red blood cells. Vitamin B2 promotes the healthy growth and respiration of all your cells, and even protects them against damage by free radicals. It helps to produce glutathione, an antioxidant that fights the free radicals leading to diseases like cancer.

Vitamin B2 is an easily absorbed, water-soluble micronutrient beneficial to all your cells;

Vitamin B2 vs. Sickle-Cell

Sickle-cell disease is a blood disorder marked by defective hemoglobin in a person's red blood cells.

Your hemoglobin carries oxygen from your lungs to the rest of your body.

The cellular support that vitamin B2 (riboflavin) provides has enabled those struck by sickle-cell to experience health improvement.

---

it even supports the production of antibodies, those cells that fight off germs and disease.

Those suffering from sickle-cell disease have shown improvement when given riboflavin.

Chemical Reactions in the Body

In this role, vitamin B2 doesn't take center stage, but it is still vital to helping our bodies use and produce other chemicals we need. For instance, vitamin B2 is needed to activate vitamin B6. It changes it into a form your body can use. It does the same for folate.

Vitamin B2 also takes an amino acid called tryptophan and changes it into another member of the vitamin B family, niacin. As you can see, vitamin B2 is an important member of your body's support team!

Good Eyesight

Studies have shown that supplementing with vitamin B2 can help prevent cataracts, those cloudy areas that develop in the lens of your eye. Cataracts impair vision and can lead to blindness.

It's important to note that in studies, riboflavin was used in conjunction with another B vitamin called niacin, so there could be some question as to which caused the cataract-fighting effect. But suffice it to say, the family of B vitamins are good for your eye health.

Headaches

Riboflavin provides good news for those who suffer from hereditary migraines. Researchers have noted that riboflavin is just as effective as prescription drugs in treating these debilitating headaches. In a three-month double-blind study, 55 migraine patients were given 400 mg of vitamin B2 regularly. Patients reported improvement after only the first month. Effectiveness increased until they hit maximum improvement at the three-month mark.[4]

What Happens When You Don't Get Enough?

When you are lacking in vitamin B2, the medical term for it is ariboflavinosis. Symptoms of deficiency in vitamin B2 include:

- Noticeable sores around the mouth
- Chapped, painful lips
- Swollen and/or purple tongue
- Inflamed eyelids
- Slow healing of wounds
- Fatigue
- Light sensitivity
- Skin rashes

There are dietary groups who can easily become riboflavin-deficient. These would include people who avoid dairy and vegans. This group should seek to get their riboflavin intake from green leafy vegetables and other sources.

People who take in low caloric amounts each day are also at risk for becoming vitamin B2 deficient. This group could include older adults and alcoholics.

Certain conditions can also put you at risk for riboflavin deficiency:

- Cataracts
- High alcohol intake
- Sickle-cell anemia
- Intestinal problems
- Chronic fatigue syndrome
- Preeclampsia (in pregnant mothers)

Food Sources

Here are the foods we can derive vitamin B2 from:

- Leafy green vegetables (especially romaine lettuce, chard, collard, and mustard greens)
- Whole grains
- Whole grain flour
- Calf's liver (has 200% daily value, so don't overeat)
- Dairy products (milk, cheese, yogurt, etc.)
- Cranberries
- Crimini mushrooms
- Asparagus
- Eggs
- Lean beef, pork, lamb

Vitamin B2 can also be found in "fortified" foods, such as:

- Baby foods
- Breakfast cereals
- Fruit drinks
- Enriched milk products
- Processed cheese
- Sauces

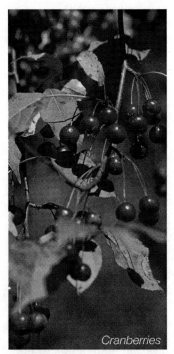
Cranberries

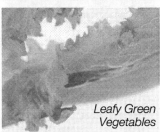
Leafy Green Vegetables

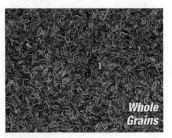
Whole Grains

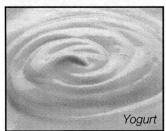
Yogurt

VITAMINS 1

Health Conditions

Vitamin B2 is useful in treating these various conditions:

- Low energy
- Low metabolism
- Cataracts
- Cancer
- Migraines
- Sickle-cell disease
- General cellular health

Dosage

Vitamin B2 or Riboflavin

Recommended Daily Intake (Men):	1-4 mg
Recommended Daily Intake (Women):	1-4 mg
Migraine Sufferers Only:	400 mg
Maximum Recommended Intake:	30 mg

Most multivitamins provide approximately 20 mg of riboflavin a day. This is perfectly fine; the extra amount is not a concern.

Possible Side Effects

There are no known safety concerns or side effects for vitamin B2 if used at recommended levels. It takes huge doses to produce side effects of both diarrhea and frequent urination. Urine will have a yellow-orange color.

Possible Interactions

Some drugs interfere with your body's ability to use riboflavin. These drugs include:

- Antidepressants
- Tetracycline
- Oral contraceptives
- AZT
- Didanosine
- Phenothiazine (psychiatric drugs)
- Antibiotics

Antibiotics cause you to shed more vitamin B2 through urination. You may want to supplement more in this case to make up for lost riboflavin.

Overusing vitamin B2 boosts your sensitivity to light. So if you are taking high doses (as a migraine sufferer would, for instance) avoid trips to the beach to avoid damage to your eyes and skin.

The Latest News

An Australian research team has discovered that by-products from bacteria that synthesize vitamin B2 or riboflavin trigger specialized immune cells in the body. They believe this will lead to greater breakthroughs in the creation of vaccines, especially for tuberculosis.

Vitamin B3 (Niacin)

What Is It For?

This vitamin has different forms, because when used as a supplement for certain therapeutic purposes, they have very distinct and different effects. Nutritionally, they are all still niacin, but each one is used for a specific therapy. There are three versions of niacin:

1. Niacin or nicotinic acid
2. Nicotinamide
3. *Inositol hexaniacinate*

The third, *Inositol hexaniacinate*, is a niacin variation that has no toxicity. Doctors recommend this supplement for those who need high amounts of niacin.

Energy and Metabolism

Like its cousins B1 and B2, B3 also helps your body convert carbohydrates, proteins, and fats into ATP, the energy molecule your cells need. This is why you can usually find these three vitamins in most multivitamins. Niacin also forms fat from carbohydrates. It also processes any alcohol that you drink.

Nicotinamide helps in the treatment of diabetes, a metabolic disorder. Global studies seek to determine if nicotinamide can delay or prevent type 1 or type 2 diabetes. Type 2 accounts for 90% of all cases of diabetes. It can also treat children's type 1 diabetes.

Cellular Support

Vitamin B3 promotes healthy skin, blood, and nerves. Used topically, gels made with nicotinamide can be helpful in treating acne.

Chemical Reactions in the Body

When the heart doesn't pump blood the way it Like other B vitamins, Niacin boosts different enzymes, triggering important chemical reactions throughout your body. It also ensures proper functioning of the digestive system.

Good Eyesight

There is evidence to show that vitamin B3 can reduce the risk of cataracts.

Cholesterol Levels

Niacin is proven to moderate your cholesterol levels, possibly as well as even the most expensive cholesterol drug on the market. It raises high-density lipoprotein (HDL, or "good" cholesterol), lowers low-density lipoprotein (LDL, or "bad" cholesterol), and lowers triglyceride levels.

In major studies, HDL was raised between 15% and 35%. LDL was lowered by five percent to 25%. Triglycerides were lowered between 20% and 50%.

Vitamin B3 can also treat atherosclerosis, the buildup of fatty deposits in your arteries.

Bone and Joint Health

Niacin can treat osteoarthritis, a degenerative joint disease in which cartilage and the underlying bone wear away. A three-month study with 72 arthritic patients included a treatment of 3,000 mg of niacin in the form of niacinamide. The patients found that their symptoms decreased by 30%.

VITAMINS 1

Brain Health

There is evidence to show that vitamin B3 can reduce the risk of Alzheimer's disease.

What Happens When You Don't Get Enough?

When you are lacking in vitamin B3, the medical term for it is pellagra. Although rare in North America, its symptoms include:

- Skin rash
- Diarrhea
- Loss of appetite
- Digestive trouble
- Mood swings
- Mental changes

Pellagra can be fatal. It was more prevalent in the southern United States during World War II. The early stages of pellagra mimic schizophrenia, so doctors would give their patients a dose of niacin. If it cured them, they knew the cause was pellagra.

People who take isoniazid (a treatment for tuberculosis) for extended periods are also at risk for becoming vitamin B3 deficient, as are alcoholics. This group includes anyone with liver problems.

Food Sources

Here are the foods we can derive vitamin B3 from:

- Peanuts and other nuts
- Seeds
- Barley
- Peas
- Eggs
- Milk
- Poultry
- Wild or brown rice
- Whole grains
- Almonds
- Lean meats
- Fish
- Organ meats

Health Conditions

Vitamin B3 is useful in treating these various conditions:

- Low energy
- Low metabolism
- Cataracts
- Atherosclerosis
- Alzheimer's
- Diabetes
- Reynaud's phenomenon
- Cholesterol

Dosage

Vitamin B3 or Niacin

Recommended Daily Intake (Men):	16 mg
Recommended Daily Intake (Women):	14 mg
Pregnant/breastfeeding Women:	19 mg
Maximum Recommended Intake:	35 mg

In the case of type 1 diabetes–prevention in young children, the recommended dosage is 25 mg daily per kilogram of body weight (1 kilogram = 2.2 pounds).

Doses to lower cholesterol and triglycerides, or to increase HDL levels are very large: one gram to four grams. Medical supervision is mandatory due to the possibility of liver damage. Your doctor will want to monitor your blood and liver regularly.

Possible Side Effects

Vitamin B3 doses of 500 mg or more should only occur under a doctor's supervision because of the heightened risk of liver damage. High doses can also cause the following:

- Diabetes
- Eye damage
- High uric acid content (which leads to gouty arthritis)

These less dangerous but nonetheless irritating side effects can occur at doses as low as 100 mg a day:

- Flushed skin
- Red rashes
- Burning, tingling, itchy sensations in face and chest
- Stomachache
- Headache

Note that all side effects listed are for supplemental niacin, not what you take in from your diet. If you need prescription niacin, there are versions that have been found to be liver-safe at high doses and that have a "sustained release" over time. The niacin version called Inositol hexaniacinate is also safer, and has not been linked with any side effects.

People who suffer from the following diseases should avoid niacin altogether unless recommended by a doctor:

- Liver disease
- Ulcers
- Gout
- Alcoholism

Possible Interactions

The form of niacin known as nicotinamide may exacerbate the effects of the following anticonvulsant medications: "Carbamazepine" and "Primidone."

There is also a slight risk that it can elevate your liver's enzyme levels and/or disrupt normal renal function when combined with statin drugs (for controlling cholesterol).

Those who take the drug isoniazid should consider supplementing

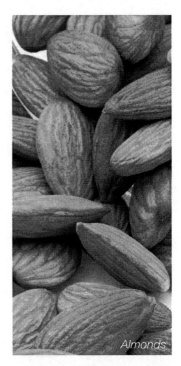

Almonds

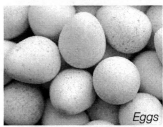

Eggs

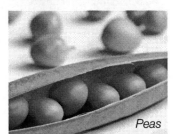

Peas

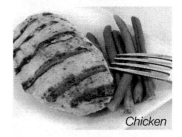

Chicken

with niacin; isoniazid interferes with the body's normal process of gaining niacin through conversion of the amino acid tryptophan.

If you take the following supplements for their antioxidant effects, they may blunt the cholesterol-controlling benefits of niacin when taken together:

- Vitamin C
- Vitamin E
- Beta-carotene
- Selenium

Finally, don't take niacin with a hot drink, as this will magnify flushing.

Reynaud's Phenomenon

Reynaud's phenomenon is a disease marked by blood vessels that restrict too much.

Niacin can stop bouts of Reynaud's by dilating the blood vessels in the arms, hands, and chest. Due to this effect, doctors now prescribe niacin for joint inflammation.

However, since niacin can cause inflammation of the liver, it should be used with caution. (See *Possible Side Effects*).

The Latest News

Two large clinical trials were conducted to see if cardiovascular health could be improved by adding niacin to statin drugs. While there were improved HDL levels, there was no heart benefit seen.

A follow-up study by researchers from the Perelman School of Medicine at the University of Pennsylvania may have found an answer. While HDL-C levels were also increased in their study, the function of the HDL to remove cholesterol from cells was not. This information will be used in new HDL therapies and studies.

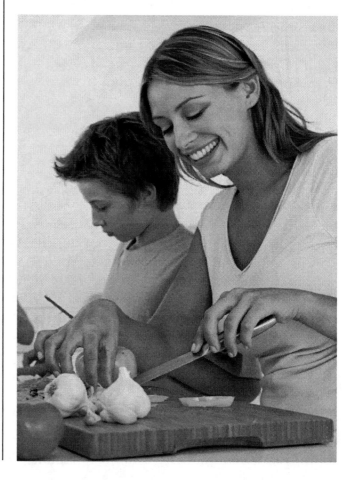

Vitamin B6

What Is It For?

This water-soluble vitamin plays a big role in many of your bodily functions and is essential for your health.

Energy and Metabolism

Your body uses more than 100 different enzymes to metabolize proteins. These proteins rely on vitamin B6. The more protein you eat, the more vitamin B6 you need.

Cellular Support

Red blood cells need vitamin B6 to be metabolized. The oxygen carrying hemoglobin in those cells can only be made with the presence of vitamin B6. Vitamin B6 also boosts hemoglobin's oxygen capacity so more oxygen is carried to your other cells.

Chemical Reactions in the Body

Vitamin B6 is essential in the creation of hormones.

B6 is also needed to convert the amino acid tryptophan into niacin (vitamin B3).

Vitamin B6 is used to form lecithin, the substance that carries fat from your system. Lecithin helps leech excess fat from the liver, and from arteries with a fatty buildup.

In tandem with vitamin B6 and folic acid, B6 helps break down the dangerous amino acid homocysteine.

Immune System

Vitamin B6 promotes white cell growth while keeping the organs that make them healthy: your lymph nodes, spleen, and thymus gland. White blood cells fight bacteria and viruses in your body.

Low levels of B6 can slow down the production of nucleic acid, another important component of your immune system.

Nervous System

Vitamin B6 is used to create and assist neurotransmitters. These are the chemical messengers that communicate information to nerve cells throughout your body. B6 also speeds up their communication, which allows your body to solve problems quicker.

Heart Health

Since vitamin B6 lowers homocysteine levels along with B12 and folic acid, it may prevent hardening of the arteries, lower blood pressure, reduce the risk of blood clots, and fend off heart disease.

Blood Sugar

When you have abnormal blood glucose levels for too long, you develop a greater risk of contracting diabetes. The enzyme that converts carbohydrates and other nutrients into glucose needs vitamin B6 to do its job. This is especially important when you're taking in low amounts of calories, causing your body to dip into its reserve energy supply to keep going.

Women's Health

Vitamin B6 can relieve bouts of morning sickness (nausea, vomiting) that women often experience during pregnancy. In one trial, 342 expectant mothers were given 30 mg of B6 or a placebo (a sugar pill or fake medication) daily. The mothers receiving B6 had fewer bouts of morning sickness than the placebo group.

One unsettled area is the effect vitamin B6 has on premenstrual syndrome (PMS). It has been beneficial for some women and not others. There is no definitive information as to B6's effectiveness in these cases.

Carpal Tunnel Syndrome

This condition is a form of arthritis brought on by repetitive motion of the wrist and hand, common in those who regularly type or use computers for extended periods. Carpal tunnel results in a squeezing of the median nerve that runs through the wrist and forearm, causing numbness, tingling, and pain in the wrist and fingers. It can become severe enough to require surgery to relieve pressure on the median nerve. Doctors believe that supplements of B6 can relieve the pain of carpal tunnel.

Brain Function

Yes, in addition to boosting memory, vitamin B6 can improve your cognitive function, actually causing you to think better!

Kidney Health

Vitamin B6 helps you avoid painful kidney stones, which are hard calcium deposits that sometimes require removal via surgery if left untreated.

What Happens When You Don't Get Enough?

Deficiency of vitamin B6 is very common. In fact, most people—probably half of the population or more—don't get enough. One reason is because vitamin B6 is one of the water-soluble vitamins; therefore, we are expelling it all the time in our waste. Taking it daily in a multivitamin or as a mixed B-vitamin supplement is a good idea.

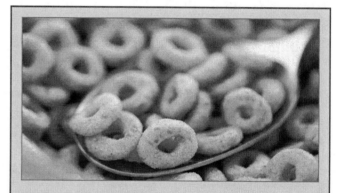

Don't Forget Breakfast

A cup of cereal each day boosts your vitamin B levels to the point where they decrease concentrations of homocysteine in the blood. When you have a vitamin B deficiency, it results in high homocysteine levels and a higher risk of vascular disease, stroke, dementia, and osteoporosis.

This was tested with 190 people aged 50–85 who weren't consuming fortified breakfast cereal or B vitamins. Their daily cup of cereal contained 440 mcg of folic acid, 1.8 mg of vitamin B6, and 4.8 mcg of vitamin B12. The result was a drop in homocysteine levels in all patients from 6.4% to 1.6%.[6]

The following symptoms could indicate a vitamin B6 deficiency:

- Skin dermatitis
- A smooth, red, or sore tongue
- Confusion
- Depression
- Weight loss
- Convulsions

Severe and continuing deficiency could bring on more serious symptoms, including:

- Diabetes
- Nervous disorders
- Heart disease
- Impairment of the immune system
- Anemia

The most at-risk groups are those with poor-quality diets, such as older adults, some children, and alcoholics. Alcohol use destroys vitamin B6 in your body. For these people, supplementing is a good idea.

Food Sources

Here are the foods we can derive vitamin B6 from:

- Organ meats
- Yeast (nutritional and brewer's)
- Wheat germ, rice, wheat bran, brown rice
- Sunflower seeds
- Legumes (especially soybeans, lentils, garbanzo beans, and lima beans)
- Walnuts (and other nuts, soybeans, seeds)
- Potatoes (with skin)
- Bananas
- Avocados
- Fortified cereal
- Lean beef, pork, and poultry
- Fish and seafood (especially clams)
- Eggs, milk, yogurt, and dairy

Health Conditions

Vitamin B6 is useful in treating these various conditions:

- Low energy
- Low metabolism
- Poor hemoglobin
- Hormone imbalance
- Arterial plaque
- Fatty liver
- Bad homocysteine levels

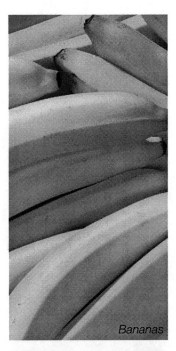

Bananas

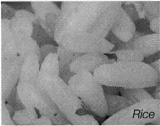

Rice

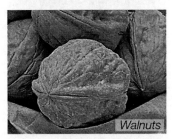

Walnuts

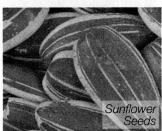

Sunflower Seeds

- Impaired immune system
- Nerve problems
- Blood pressure problems
- Heart disease
- Abnormal blood sugar
- Diabetes
- Morning sickness
- Carpal tunnel syndrome
- Poor memory, difficulty thinking
- Kidney stones
- Children's asthma
- Children's autism

Dosage

Vitamin B6

Recommended Daily Intake (Men):	1.3 mg
Recommended Daily Intake (Men, over 50):	1.7 mg
Recommended Daily Intake (Women):	1.3 mg
Pregnant/breastfeeding Women:	2.0 mg
Maximum Recommended Intake:	50 mg

For higher doses, you should first consult your doctor.

The best way to take vitamin B6 is in the form of a multivitamin or a B-complex supplement, since it works hand-in-hand with its vitamin-B cousins.

Possible Side Effects

Side effects usually occur only in very high doses of B6, meaning about 500–1,000 mg a day. These doses can cause the following:

- Nerve damage (sensory neuropathy)
- Numbness in the extremities
- Difficulty walking
- Severe acne

Possible Interactions

Doses of 5 mg or more of vitamin B6 can interfere with the drug levodopa.

Conversely, there are drugs that can inhibit your body's absorption of vitamin B6. These include:

- Isoniazid (for treating tuberculosis)
- L-DOPA (for neurological impairments and Parkinson's disease)
- Theophylline (a children's asthma drug)
- In these cases, consult a doctor on taking vitamin B6 supplements.

The Latest News

A 2012 study in the *Journal of Nutrition* shows a strong connection between chronic inflammation and vitamin B6. Those involved in the test showed the lowest levels of inflammation when high levels of vitamin B6 were present. Chronic inflammation is an emerging risk factor for diseases such as type 2 diabetes, heart disease, and stroke.

Vitamin B9 (Folic Acid)

What Is It For?

Vitamin B9, or folic acid, is absolutely essential for many bodily functions, including cell division, creation of new cells, and maintenance of your current cells. Keep in mind that you'll rarely ever see "vitamin B9" used for labeling purposes. Rather, you will see the words "folic acid" or "folate" substituted. Folate is the synthetic form of folic acid that goes into foods that are fortified with this vitamin. In spite of the slight confusion in names, folic acid is still part of the water-soluble vitamin-B family.

Cellular Support

Your cells need adequate amounts of folate to divide properly. Folate also helps create and maintain new cells. This is why folic acid is so important for expectant mothers, newborns, and infants. In these children, cells and tissue are growing and regenerating at accelerated rates. The immune cells need the support of folic acid. Folic acid also creates healthy red blood cells, thereby eliminating anemia.

The building blocks of our bodies, DNA and RNA, both depend heavily on folic acid. The cellular structure of our DNA is where your genetic information is stored. RNA controls the formulation of protein in your cells. Folic acid protects your DNA from changes that can lead to cancer when a cell mutates.

Chemical Reactions in the Body

When homocysteine levels in your body get too high, it can lead to heart disease and stroke. Folic acid breaks down this dangerous amino acid, transforming it into methionine that the body can then use.

Heart Health

Folic acid is a great way to prevent heart disease. Independent studies have shown that folic acid can cut your risk of cardiovascular disease in half!

Women's Health

Doctors recommend folic acid for pregnant women, since it cuts the risk of birth defects by 50%–80%.

Mood

For those suffering from depression, folate has proven itself a useful tool. If you battle major depression and are taking SSRI antidepressants, folate actually increases the effectiveness of those medicines.

Cancer

Because of folic acid's effectiveness on the cellular level, it is widely thought that it can prevent certain cancers. Many studies have shown that a lack of folate may predispose you to the following cancers:

- Lung
- Colon
- Liver

- Oral cavity
- Breast
- Pancreas
- Cervix

This has been found especially true for colon cancer. Huge observational studies found that supplementing with folic acid over a long period of time helps you avoid colon cancer.[7]

What Happens When You Don't Get Enough?

As we've alluded to before, pregnant women should make sure their folic acid levels are good, to prevent low birth weight in their babies, as well as to reduce the risk of neural tube defects.

Lack of folate is associated with a higher number of pre-cancerous polyps in the colon, which raises the risk for colorectal cancer.

The following symptoms could indicate a vitamin B9 deficiency:

- Overall weakness
- Smooth, red, or sore tongue
- Heart palpitations
- Shortness of breath
- Irritability
- Forgetfulness
- Headaches
- Behavioral disorders

The most at-risk groups are the following:

- Pregnant women
- Alcohol abusers
- Liver disease patients
- Those with malabsorption problems
- Kidney dialysis patients

Talk with your doctor about whether supplementing with folic acid could be a good option for you.

Food Sources

Here are the foods we can derive folic acid from:

- Leafy green vegetables (especially spinach)
- Fruits (especially citrus)
- Legumes (especially lentils and chickpeas)
- Great northern beans
- Long-grain rice
- Green peas
- Peanuts
- Oranges, orange juice
- Romaine lettuce
- Liver
- Fortified breakfast cereal
- Asparagus
- Celery
- Beets
- Baked beans
- Broccoli
- Avocados
- Wheat germ
- Tomato juice

Health Conditions

Folic acid is useful in treating these various conditions:

- Cancer
- Birth defects
- Poor hemoglobin
- Heart disease
- Bad homocysteine levels
- Impaired immune system
- Anemia
- Blood pressure problems
- Stroke
- Depression
- Poor memory, difficulty thinking

Dosage

Vitamin B9, Folic Acid, Folate

For higher doses, you should first consult your doctor.

Possible Side Effects

Recommended Daily Intake (Men):	400 mcg
Recommended Daily Intake (Women):	400 mcg
Pregnant/breastfeeding WVTlomen:	
600 mcg	
Maximum Recommended Intake: 1,000 mcg	

Since it's water-soluble, there is no danger in getting your folic acid from food items.

Side effects usually occur only in very high doses of B9, around 5–15 mg a day. These doses can cause the following:

- Upset stomach
- Diarrhea
- Rash
- Altered sleep patterns
- Vivid dreams
- Impaired judgment
- Psychosis
- Zinc depletion

Epileptics and those taking anticonvulsants may experience an increase in seizures due to folic acid intake.

Possible Interactions

Although uncommon, folic acid supplementation can mask a deficiency in vitamin B12. A B12 deficiency can lead to permanent nerve damage. However, the body does need folic acid in order to use vitamin B12. So if you are over 50, you should have a doctor check your B12 levels before you embark on supplementation with folic acid.

A positive interaction has been discovered that can benefit sufferers of arthritis and psoriasis. Folic acid can reduce the side effects of the drug methotrexate when the two are taken simultaneously.

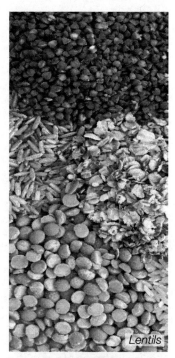

Lentils

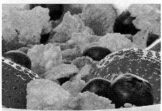

Oranges

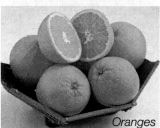

Fortified Breakfast Cereal

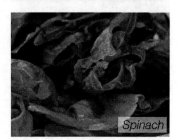

Spinach

Doses of vitamin B9 can interfere with the drugs phenytoin and primidone.[8]

Conversely, there are drugs that can inhibit your body's absorption of vitamin B9. These include:

- Antacids
- H-2 blockers
- Metformin (a diabetic drug)
- Diuretics
- Nitric oxide
- Bile acid sequestrants
- Anticonvulsant medication

- Sulfasalazine (colon therapy)
- Barbiturates
- Pancreatin

In these cases, consult a doctor before taking vitamin B9 supplements.

The Latest News

A new study from the UC Davis MIND Institute suggests that women who take folic acid supplements during the first month of pregnancy reduce the risk of childhood autism. The recommended dose was 600 mcg daily.

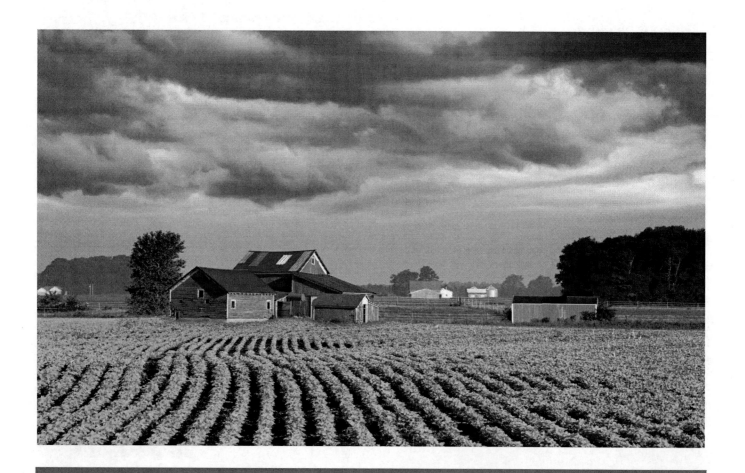

Vitamin B12

What Is It For?

As opposed to other members of the vitamin B family, B12 is more of a background player, supporting its vitamin-B cousins. While B12 has been recommended for treating a number of diseases, the medical evidence is not conclusive enough to suggest supplementing with it for those reasons.

Medical researchers are still trying to determine B12's effectiveness when it comes to treating:

- Male infertility
- Alzheimer's disease
- Asthma
- HIV
- Multiple sclerosis
- Restless legs syndrome
- Tinnitus
- Blotchy skin
- Depression
- Osteoporosis
- Periodontal disease

As such, supplementation with vitamin B12 for these particular conditions may or may not provide benefits.

Here is what B12 has been shown effective for:

Cellular Support

As with folic acid, B12 works to ensure that your red blood cells are properly formed and that your cells divide the way they should. When you're growing and developing, cells divide more rapidly, and vitamin B12 is key to that function. This is especially true for the areas of your body that have a high turnover of cells—your intestines and blood.

Like folic acid, B12 can help to rapidly make DNA while protecting your cells from the dangerous mutations that can lead to cancer.

Chemical Reactions in the Body

When homocysteine levels in your body get too high, it can lead to heart disease and stroke. Just like other B vitamins and folic acid, B12 breaks down this dangerous amino acid, transforming it into methionine that the body can then use.

Vitamin B12 also helps your body create *S-adenosylmethionine*, an important detoxifying agent.

Heart Health

By bringing down your homocysteine levels, B12 helps you avoid the risk of heart disease.

Immune System

Vitamin B12 ensures that your body can respond quickly to infections.

Nervous System

A fatty sheath made of a complex protein called myelin protects each of your nerves. Vitamin B12 metabolizes the fatty acids that are crucial to maintaining this protective covering. When you are deficient in vitamin B12 for too long, you risk nerve degeneration.

Cancer

Vitamin B12 helps your body create antioxidants, which fight cancer.

Brain Health

Vitamin B12 is used to create chemicals that your brain uses for healthy functioning.

Joint Health

B12 assists in the creation of tissues in your joints.

Stomach Acid

B12 can enhance the effects of drugs that are meant to lower stomach acid.

What Happens When You Don't Get Enough?

Vegans and those avoiding meat always have to be on guard against B12 deficiency. This group tends to avoid dairy products and eggs. Their deficiency doesn't occur overnight, but it will start to take its toll after years of this type of dietary lifestyle. However, there are also sufferers who simply have a problem absorbing this vitamin.

For your system to absorb it, vitamin B12 needs to combine with a protein that is found in your digestive juices. Some people don't make enough of this protein for absorption of B12 to take place. This is usually true of older adults and people who are on low-protein diets.

The following symptoms could indicate a vitamin B12 deficiency:

- Fatigue
- Menstrual problems
- Listless feeling
- Shortness of breath
- Sore tongue
- Forgetfulness
- Loss of balance
- Disorientation
- Depression and/or anxiety
- Numbness/tingling in the hands or feet
- Poor resistance to infection

Food Sources

Since vitamin B12 is found mainly in meat, eggs, and dairy, there are two groups that may definitely need to supplement their diet: vegetarians and vegans. This is why most vegan products for sale are fortified with B12.

Here are the foods we can derive vitamin B12 from:

- Free-range eggs
- Organ meats (liver, kidney)
- Lamb
- Cheese
- Beef
- Clams
- Milk

Some of the fortified foods that have been B12-enhanced include:

- Veggie burgers
- Textured vegetable protein
- Soy milk
- Margarine
- Breakfast cereals

Health Conditions

Vitamin B12 is useful in treating these various conditions:

- Cancer
- Nerve damage
- Poor hemoglobin
- Heart disease
- Bad homocysteine levels
- Impaired immune system
- Anemia
- Joint problems
- High stomach acid
- Depression
- Poor memory, difficulty thinking
- Fatigue
- Anxiety
- Loss of balance

Dosage

You will usually find vitamin B12 in formulations that include vitamins B1, B2, B3, B5 (pantothenic acid), and folic acid. Check labels to be sure B12 is present.

Vitamin B12

Recommended Daily Intake (Men):	2.4–3 mcg
Recommended Daily Intake (Women):	2.4–3 mcg
Anemia Sufferers:	1,000 mcg
Maximum Recommended Intake:	1,000 mcg

Most people don't need much B12 daily, but those with anemia or those who suffer from high homocysteine levels will want to take more. People in the latter group should take at least 500 mcg together with 0.5–5 mg of folic acid and 16 mg of pyridoxine. This has shown to be a successful combination.

In the case of anemia sufferers, you will want to consult your doctor before supplementing with vitamin B12.

Possible Side Effects

Vitamin B12 is very safe, even in large doses. There is little danger of toxicity, but those with acne should be aware that large doses of B12 could make acne worse. Pregnant women and children can feel completely safe taking this nutrient.

Possible Interactions

There are no known interactions with vitamin B12 that you should be concerned about.

However, there are drugs that can inhibit your body's absorption of vitamin B12. If you are taking any on this list, you should consider supplementing to avoid B12 deficiency. These drugs include:

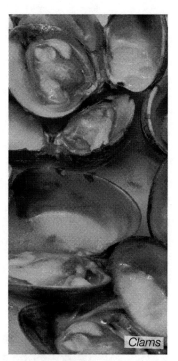

Clams

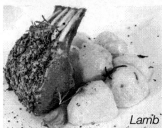

Lamb

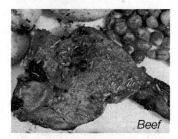

Beef

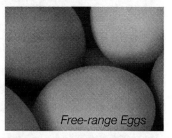

Free-range Eggs

- Proton pump inhibitors
- H-2 blockers
- Colchicine
- Metformin
- Nitrous oxide
- Supplemental potassium
- Antiseizure medications
- Phenformin
- Zidovudine (AZT, Combivin, Retrovin)
- Antibiotics

In these cases, consult a doctor before taking vitamin B12 supplements.

The Latest News

Results from a seven-year Finnish study were published in the October 19, 2010 issue of *Neurology*, the publication of the *American Academy of Neurology*. It looked at 271 people aged 65-79 who didn't have dementia at the beginning of the study. Over the time period, 17 people developed Alzheimer's disease. The blood of the entire group was tested, and those with higher levels of vitamin B12 had reduced their risk of Alzheimer's.

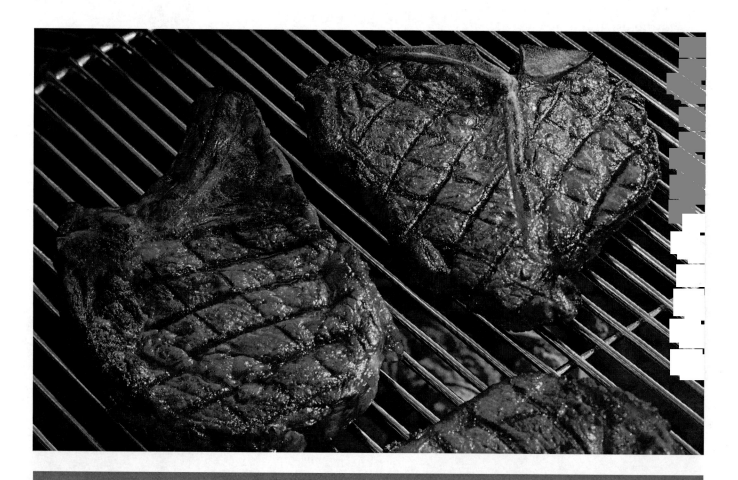

Vitamin C

What Is It For?

Vitamin C is a strong, water-soluble nutrient that tackles a whole host of diseases and infections. The main ones are listed here, but it has been suggested by many professionals that vitamin C may impact many, many more. A lot of evidence on C versus these other diseases is still questionable, but since the vitamin is so safe to use, there's no real reason to think that it wouldn't be beneficial.

Medical researchers are still trying to determine vitamin C's effectiveness when it comes to treating:

- Gallbladder disease
- Dementia
- Bipolar disorder
- Migraines
- Parkinson's disease
- Heart disease
- Osteoarthritis
- Allergies
- Periodontal disease
- Rheumatoid arthritis
- Hepatitis
- Menopausal symptoms
- HIV
- Cervical dysplasia

Here is what vitamin C has been shown effective for:

Cellular Support

Vitamin C is the primary antioxidant in your body. Also known as ascorbic acid, vitamin C not only protects the outside of cells from free radical damage, but the interior cellular structure too. The oxidation from free radicals can lead to many severe diseases, including cancer.

When combined with vitamin E, it results in a powerful antioxidant that fights free radicals. Vitamin C works in the body's water while E works in the body's fat, making an effective team.

Chemical Reactions in the Body

Your body uses vitamin C to build collagen, the most important protein you manufacture. Collagen holds your connective tissues in place, essentially holding your body together. Vitamin C creates an even stronger structure by allowing connective fibers to cross-weave over themselves like a basket.

When there is a lack of vitamin C, this cross-linking doesn't take place, resulting in scurvy-like conditions. Teeth begin to loosen within your gums and blood vessels can break down beneath the surface of your skin.

Vitamin C also helps your body absorb iron.

Energy and Metabolism

Vitamin C is used to create a compound in your body known as carnitine. Carnitine carries fatty acids into your cells to provide them with energy. That's why a lack of vitamin C can leave you feeling fatigued.

VITAMINS 1

It's essential that your body get enough vitamin C for the metabolism of cholesterol, fats, and certain proteins.

Immune System

Vitamin C is vital to a healthy, well-functioning immune system. A study from the 60th meeting of the American Academy of Allergy, Asthma and Immunology showed that people who took C supplements daily did indeed boost their immune systems. Texas researchers wanted to know if vitamin C could increase protection from viral infections. They gave the participants one gram of vitamin C a day, then watched immune cells and recorded any changes. After two weeks of supplementation, the results were as follows:

- Higher levels of natural killer cells in the bloodstream

- More activated T cells

- T cells that produced far more antiviral compounds and less compounds that attack the flu virus

It's apparent that vitamin C significantly increases your body's immunity to viruses. Vitamin C helps your body release interferon. This is a virus-fighting antibody that wraps around the outside of cells, keeping viruses like the flu from attaching themselves and spreading.

Vitamin C also boosts and creates more of your body's primary infection-fighters, namely white blood cells. It's a crucial component in the healing of wounds and bone fractures as well.

The common cold is one infection that vitamin C seems to be made for. A cold is essentially an upper respiratory tract infection. Large doses of vitamin C (up to 1,000 mg a day) can reduce cold symptoms, and eliminate the infection more rapidly.

Vitamin C has been shown to reduce the risk of contracting a respiratory infection after strenuous endurance exercise. In fact, one study gave 92 cross-country runners 600 mg of vitamin C daily for three weeks right before a race. The researchers charted the difference in sickness between those getting the vitamin and those who were given placebo pills. Two weeks after the race, about 70% of the placebo group developed cold-like symptoms. Of the vitamin C group, only 33% developed cold symptoms.[10]

Eye Health

As opposed to getting vitamin C through diet, it appears that long-term vitamin C supplementation can help strengthen your eyes in addition to preventing the free radicals that give you cataracts.

This is especially true for diabetics, because vitamin C reduces the buildup of sorbitol in their cells. Sorbitol is a sugar alcohol that can get trapped in the cells of the retina, the cells of the lens, and the associated nerves, leading to damage later on.

Macular degeneration is the second-most common cause of eye injury. It's a progressive disease of the retina resulting in blurred central vision, and eventual blindness. Vitamin C supplements may be able to not just prevent it, but also halt it once it's begun.

Blood Pressure

While it doesn't lower it by huge amounts, vitamin C does indeed decrease blood pressure. However, vitamin C protects your liver and kidneys from damage due to hypertension, which is why many doctors prescribe the supplement for sufferers or those who are at risk for hypertension.

Recovery from Injuries

Arm and leg injuries can have lingering effects, such as pain, swelling, movement problems, and difficulty in healing. These are symptoms of a condition known as reflex sympathetic dystrophy, or RSD. Vitamin C has shown impressive results in eliminating RSD. In a study of 123 people recovering from wrist fractures, some were given 500 mg of vitamin C daily; some were given a placebo. After 50 days, the C group had significantly fewer cases of RSD than the placebo group.

Vitamin C will also reduce your tendency to bruise easily.

Women's Health

Pregnant women can reduce the risk of the dangerous condition known as preeclampsia by supplementing with vitamin C.

What Happens When You Don't Get Enough?

Although it's not seen very much today, a vitamin C deficiency can result in a disease called scurvy. Symptoms include anemia, gum disease (painful, receding, and bleeding gums), and skin hemorrhaging (also called "blood spots," these occur just under the surface). The most at-risk for scurvy are malnourished people and alcoholics.

The following symptoms could indicate a vitamin C deficiency:

- Bleeding gums
- Bruising easily
- Slow healing of wounds
- Dry hair
- Nosebleeds
- Fatigue
- Weakened immune system
- Rough, dry skin
- Split ends

Since it's water-soluble, it's easy to lose vitamin C through urination. That's one reason why supplementation is such a good idea.

Food Sources

There are a lot of great sources for vitamin C, both in fruits and vegetables. The abundance of choices means that anyone should be able to easily find a dietary source of vitamin C they like.

Here are the fruits we can derive vitamin C from:

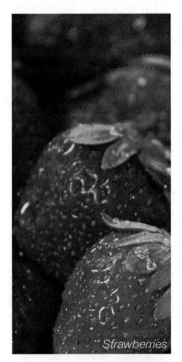
Strawberries

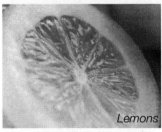
Lemons

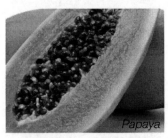
Papaya

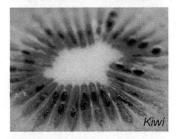
Kiwi

- Strawberries
- Oranges
- Lemons
- Papayas
- Watermelon
- Kiwi
- Cantaloupe
- Grapefruit
- Tomatoes
- Pineapple

Some of the vegetables that have vitamin C:

- Red peppers, green peppers
- Broccoli
- Cauliflower
- Asparagus
- Brussels sprouts
- Mustard greens
- Romaine lettuce
- Kale
- Cabbage
- Spinach
- Collard greens
- Fennel

Health Conditions

Vitamin C is useful in treating these various conditions:

- Cancer
- Lack of collagen
- Scurvy
- Fatigue
- High cholesterol
- Impaired immune system
- Common cold
- Influenza
- Viral infections
- White blood cell count
- Cataracts
- Macular degeneration
- Diabetes
- High blood pressure
- Reflex sympathetic dystrophy
- Preeclampsia

Dosage

Vitamin C can be taken safely at high doses. This is especially good news for those trying to prevent colds or recovering from colds. When supplementing for this purpose, you should space your intake throughout the day, rather than taking it all at once. This will keep you from losing it all through urination, as you would if you took one big dose.

Vitamin C

Recommended Daily Intake (Men):	500-3,000 mg
Recommended Daily Intake (Women):	500-3,000 mg
Maximum Recommended Intake:	2,000 mcg

Possible Side Effects

Vitamin C is very safe, even in prolonged doses. There is little danger of toxicity, but those with kidney or liver disease should be careful, since a maximum safe dosage for vitamin C has not been determined.

Temporary diarrhea can be a side effect that usually goes away once your body gets used to the vitamin C intake.

Vitamin C doses of one gram or more daily can result in kidney stones or deep vein thrombosis.

Possible Interactions

Do not combine high amounts of vitamin C with high doses of "Tylenol," as it raises the risk of liver damage.

High doses of vitamin C (three grams or more) may impair your body's absorption of copper and iron.

Doses like these can also reduce the effectiveness of warfarin or heparin.

Vitamin C may interact with the following drugs:

- Estradiol
- Fluphenazine
- Statin drugs
- Protease inhibitors
- Salsalate

In these cases, consult a doctor on taking vitamin C supplements.

You may need more vitamin C if you take the following:

- Aspirin
- Anti-inflammatory drugs
- Oral contraceptives

Again, in these cases, you should check with your doctor.

The Latest News

The 2011 issue of the *Journal of Biological Chemistry* featured a study by Lund University researchers that discovered an exciting new use for vitamin C. It may be a viable treatment for Alzheimer's disease. It appears that vitamin C dissolves lumps consisting of toxic protein plaques that cause nerve cell damage in the brain. These lumps usually attack the memory centers of the brain first. The findings have opened up new possibilities in Alzheimer's research.

The Vitamin One-Two Punch for Prostate Cancer

The team of vitamins C and E can help knockout prostate cancer.

A 2004 study by three researchers showed that the vitamin combo stunted the growth of non-responsive human prostate cancer cells.

The cell was reduced from four percent on the small end, to a whopping 83% on the high end.

These two tough fighters obviously can be key in taking down this deadly cancer.[9]

VITAMINS 1

Vitamin D

What Is It For?

Here is what vitamin D has been shown effective for:

Cellular Support

It's believed that vitamin D promotes cellular health, or cell differentiation. Simply put, it promotes healthy growth in cells that are developing properly, and disrupts abnormal growth (malignant cells) that can develop into cancers.

Due to this property of cell differentiation, vitamin D may be a good treatment against cancer. Information is still forthcoming, and there has been mixed results in this area. However, vitamin D may have a role in reducing these cancers:

- Skin cancer
- Breast cancer
- Colon cancer
- Pancreatic cancer
- Prostate cancer

Chemical Reactions in the Body

Your body uses vitamin D to absorb calcium from the food you eat. Vitamin D is also a hormone. It's synthesized when our skin is exposed to sunlight. In fact, sunlight is the best source of vitamin D.

Vitamin D may also reduce the risk of getting type 1 diabetes.

Bone Health

When you have high levels of calcium and phosphorus in your bloodstream, your body uses it to harden or build up your bones. Without it, you can develop rickets or osteoporosis.

There is good evidence to show that vitamin D can prevent this bone-crippling disease in older adults and especially women. Women with low levels of vitamin D do experience osteoporosis. However, supplementing with a combination of vitamin D and calcium can slow it down and, in some cases, reverse it.

Another benefit of this kind of supplementation is an increase in bone density, making you less prone to breaks and bone fractures.

Skin Health

Vitamin D has been a long-standing treatment for psoriasis in the form of calcipotriol. Although it sounds like calcium, this form of vitamin D actually has nothing to do with it. Calcipotriol is for topical use, and applying it to the skin has shown some success.

Women's Health

Supplementing with vitamin D and calcium may help women who suffer polycystic ovary syndrome.

What Happens When You Don't Get Enough?

Although it's not seen very much today, a vitamin D deficiency can result in a disease called rickets. The name comes from the Old English word "wrikken," which means to twist or bend. This describes the bone deformities that can occur with rickets, as it softens the bones and makes them prone to fractures. Although primarily a children's disease, adults can suffer it as well.

Since sunlight is the primary source of vitamin D, it's logical that people who live in northern latitudes could experience deficiencies, especially the elderly. Because prolonged sun exposure can also be damaging and raise your risk for skin cancer, many choose to supplement their diet instead.

Cultures that consume a lot of fatty fish have an advantage over the rest of us, as they are taking in good amounts of vitamin D. You can get it through milk, but you have to make sure it has been fortified with D.

The following symptoms could indicate a vitamin D deficiency:

- Osteoporosis
- Muscle cramps
- Twitches

Those over 50 should make sure they are getting some vitamin D each day.

Food Sources

Here are the foods we can derive vitamin D from:

- Liver
- Enriched milk and dairy products
- Fatty fish (mackerel, salmon, tuna, halibut, cod)
- Eggs
- Fortified bread
- Fortified breakfast cereal
- Shrimp

Health Conditions

Vitamin D is useful in treating these various conditions:

- Cancer
- Osteoporosis
- Rickets
- Type 1 diabetes
- Psoriasis
- Polycystic ovary syndrome
- Muscle cramps
- Twitches

Dosage

Vitamin D can be taken safely at suggested doses; extremely high doses can result in toxicity.

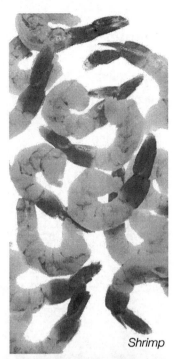

Shrimp

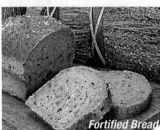

Fortified Bread

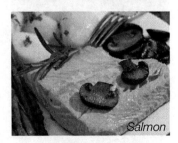

Salmon

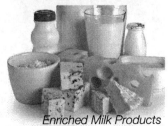

Enriched Milk Products

VITAMINS 1

Vitamin D

Recommended Daily Intake (Men):	200 IU (5 mcg)
Recommended Daily Intake (Women):	200 IU (5 mcg)
Recommended Daily Intake (Men 51 and older):	400 IU (10 mcg)
Recommended Daily Intake (Women 51 and older):	400 IU (10 mcg)
Recommended Daily Intake (Men 71 and older):	600 IU (15 mcg)
Recommended Daily Intake (Women 71 and older):	600 IU (15 mcg)
Pregnant and Nursing Women:	200 IU
Maximum Recommended Intake:	2,000 mcg

Possible Side Effects

There is no definitive information on what constitutes an extremely high dose of vitamin D, one that would bring on toxicity. Common sense dictates that if you supplement with D daily in high doses (1,000 IU a day, for example) for an extended period of time (six months), you will experience toxicity. This is because the level of calcium in your blood will be too high. It's best to stick to the recommended daily levels.

Symptoms of toxicity can include:

- Weakness
- Dry mouth
- Nausea

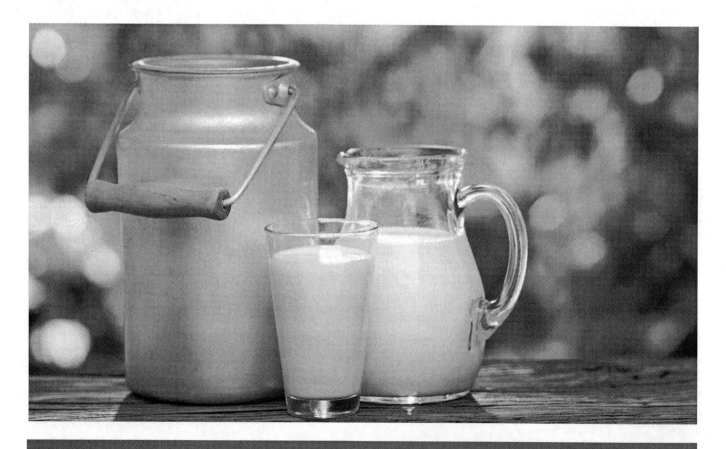

- Vomiting
- Abdominal cramps
- Bone pain
- Irritability
- Dizziness

Possible Interactions

If you suffer from sarcoidosis or hyperparathyroidism, do not take vitamin D unless specifically ordered to by your doctor.

Women with osteoporosis need to supplement with vitamin D. Be aware that if you take thiazide diuretics, combining them with D and calcium raises your risk of hypercalcemia.

Vitamin D vs. Prostate Cancer

Epidemiological research has shown a link between decreased vitamin D levels and prostate cancer risk.

This prompted a study by researchers Stewart and Weigel from the Baylor College of Medicine in Houston, Texas. They found that vitamin D reduces the growth of cancer cells, particularly prostate cancer cells.

They believe these results merit further study into vitamin D's role as a prostate cancer treatment.[11]

Certain drugs can interfere with the absorption or activity of vitamin D. You may need more vitamin D if you take the following:

- Calcium channel blockers
- Phenobarbital
- Phenytoin
- Cimetidine
- Isoniazid
- Primidone
- Stimulant laxatives
- Valproic acid
- Corticosteroids
- Heparin
- Rifampin
- Vitamin A

The Latest News

A recent study has discovered a link between vitamin D and daytime sleepiness. The study also discovered that race plays an important factor. It looked at 81 sleep clinic patients who were diagnosed with sleep disorders. After blood tests, it was discovered that a correlation exists between low vitamin D levels and excessive daytime sleepiness. It was not unusual to find this more prevalent in blacks, since one of the risk factors for low vitamin D is increased skin pigmentation. The results were published in the December 15, 2012 issue of the *Journal of Clinical Sleep Medicine.*

VITAMINS 1

Vitamin E

What Is It For?

Vitamin E may be the most important weapon in your health arsenal due to the scope of what it can treat. It's a critical antioxidant in the fats and oils of your body. Vitamin C works in tandem with vitamin E in the water of your body to combat free radicals. Taking both vitamins provides a one-two antioxidant punch.

Here is what vitamin E has been shown effective for:

Cellular Support

Like vitamin D, vitamin E controls cell division and regulates blood cells. It also promotes the growth of connective tissue and fights inflammation.

Since vitamin E also promotes healthy cells and has powerful antioxidant properties, it may be a good treatment against cancer. Information is still forthcoming on the total scope of cancers for which this vitamin is effective; however, vitamin E may have a role in reducing these cancers:

- Mouth cancer
- Throat cancer
- Liver cancer
- Lung cancer
- Colon cancer

Immune System

When combined with vitamin C, vitamin E becomes a powerful flu fighter. Vitamin E's regulation of your cells stimulates the production of the immune cells that kill invading viruses and bacteria.

Vitamin E can reverse the decline of your immune system as you age. In this regard, vitamin E is very important to older adults who become more susceptible to flu, sometimes leading to pneumonia. A double-blind study backs this claim. Eighty-eight people over 65 years old were given either vitamin E or a placebo. The participants were then vaccinated against hepatitis B, pneumonia, and tetanus. Their immune responses were then examined. Those who received vitamin E produced vastly greater amounts of antibodies than the placebo group. They also experienced 30% fewer infections.

The consensus for older adults is that supplementing with vitamin E will not only enhance the immune system and raise the levels of infection-fighting cells, but it will also reverse a declining immune system. The theory is that since immune cells are constantly changing and synthesizing bodily material as they grow, vitamin E could ensure that new, strong, and healthy molecules replace the older, damaged ones that hamper your immune system. Vitamin E also reduces the production of suppressor or T cells, thus keeping your immune system at its highest level of effectiveness.

A one-year study, published by the *Journal of the American Medical Association* (*JAMA*) looked at vitamin E's ability to prevent respiratory tract infections in nursing home residents. The researchers wanted to see if vitamin E improved immune response. They wrote, "We observed a protective effect of vitamin E supplementation on upper respiratory tract infections, particularly the common cold, that merits further investigation."

Blood Sugar

Vitamin E appears to support your body's ability to produce glucose. As such, it may be useful in the prevention and treatment of diabetes.

Heart Health

Your cardiac system gets a boost from vitamin E.

Nervous System

It's thought that, because vitamin E is so good in fighting free radicals, it may limit neurological impairments. Your nerve cells are highly susceptible to free radical damage.

Memory and Brain Function

Vitamin E helps limit the symptoms of Alzheimer's disease, as well as treating dementia.

What Happens When You Don't Get Enough?

Your diet would have to be very poor for you to become dangerously deficient in vitamin E.

Minor deficiencies are more common, mainly in those who have difficulty absorbing dietary fat, or those who have disorders that inhibit the body's ability to metabolize fat (celiac disease). This kind of deficiency can go unnoticed for a long time, usually only detected when nerve tissue damage occurs, characterized by lowered cognitive skills. Once a minor deficiency becomes a major one, the damage can be irreversible.

Food Sources

When buying natural vitamin E for supplementation, look for "mixed tocopherols." Natural ones will appear on labels as "d-alpha," "d-gamma," "d-delta," and "d-beta" tocopherol.

Here are the foods we can derive vitamin E from:

- Polyunsaturated vegetable oils
- Whole grains
- Broccoli
- Olives
- Parsley

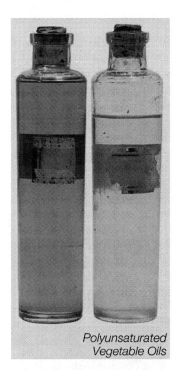
Polyunsaturated Vegetable Oils

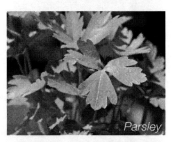
Lobster

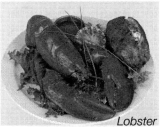
Parsley

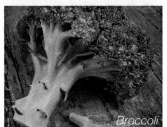
Broccoli

- Salmon, tuna, shrimp, lobster
- Avocados
- Seeds and nuts (especially sunflower seeds, peanuts, almonds)
- Leafy greens (mustard greens, collard greens, spinach, kale)
- Turnip
- Papaya
- Egg yolks

Health Conditions

Vitamin E is useful in treating these various conditions:

- Cancer
- Inflammation
- Influenza
- Viruses and bacteria
- Impaired immune system
- Respiratory tract infection
- Common cold
- Pneumonia
- Diabetes
- Impaired cardiac function
- Nerve damage
- Alzheimer's disease
- Cognitive function
- Memory
- Dementia

Dosage

Vitamin E can be taken safely at suggested doses for different forms, listed here:

Vitamin E

Recommended Daily Intake (Men):	15 mg
Recommended Daily Intake (Women):	15 mg
Recommended Intake (Pregnant Women):	19 mg

Therapeutic doses:

Recommended Daily Intake (synthetic E):	50-80 mg
Recommended Daily Intake (natural E):	25-400 mg
Maximum Recommended Intake:	1,000 mg

Possible Side Effects

Side effects with vitamin E are rare. Even elderly people taking 530 mg daily for extended periods experienced no negative impacts of any kind. This was tested up to four months.

That being said, prolonged use at high doses for longer stretches has not been investigated, so it would be prudent to limit intake for the sake of caution.

Vitamin E is an anticoagulant, which can result in bleeding problems if taken in very high levels.

Possible Interactions

Care must be taken when combining vitamin E with certain herbs like garlic and *Gingko biloba*, because it can cause blood-thinning problems.

At high doses, vitamin E can exert an antiplatelet effect, increasing the risk of stroke.

Certain drugs and medical situations merit caution with supplementation of vitamin E. It is extremely important to consult with your doctor if you are:

- Taking anticoagulants
- Taking antiplatelets
- Taking chemotherapy drugs
- Taking medications to control blood sugar levels
- Suffering from blood disorders
- About to have surgery
- About to give birth

Vitamin E vs. Prostate Cancer

Vitamin E has had significant results fighting prostate cancer.

In one study, 30,000 male smokers were given 50 mg of vitamin E daily for five to eight years. Results showed a 32% drop in the incidence of prostate cancer, and a 41% drop in prostate cancer deaths.

This is especially startling considering that the men in the study were active smokers, which greatly increases the risk for cancer.[12]

The Latest News

New information on vitamin E indicates that specific forms, gamma and delta tocopherols, are more beneficial in preventing colon, lung, breast, and prostate cancers than forms such as alpha tocopherols. This was the finding of a 2012 study by scientists at the Center for Cancer Prevention Research at Rutgers Ernest Mario School of Pharmacy, and the Cancer Institute of New Jersey. These forms of vitamin E are found in soybean, canola, and corn oils.

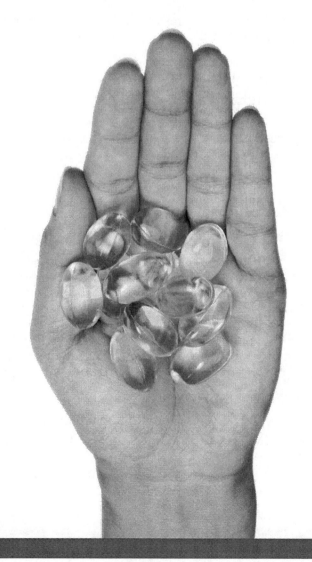

VITAMINS 1

Vitamin K

What Is It For?

Vitamin K is a different kind of vitamin. It's actually produced by our intestinal bacteria! This version of vitamin K is referred as "K-2." "K-1" is the designation for the vitamin K found in food, and "K-3" is the synthetic form created in the laboratory, and available to patients only through prescription.

Here is what vitamin K has been shown effective for:

Cellular Support

As with other vitamins like D and E, vitamin K may promote healthy cells by controlling cell growth. Since it may be able to control the growth of mutated cells as well as healthy ones, vitamin K could be yet another cancer fighter.

Chemical Reactions in the Body

In order to promote healthy blood clotting, vitamin K sets off a number of chemical reactions to bring about this result: your body uses the vitamin K in your system to produce prothrombin, which is then converted to thrombin. The thrombin then turns the chemical fibrinogen into fibrin, which then creates the blood clot. This is how our body keeps internal and external wounds from bleeding excessively.

It is this chemical reaction that enabled us to discover vitamin K in the first place. Vitamin K

is one of the fat-soluble vitamins that get stored in your tissues.

Bone Health

Vitamin K helps to form new bone by "gluing" calcium to it. It may also keep you from losing excessive amounts of calcium in your urine.

This could be good news for those with osteoporosis. The bone weakening effect of this disease makes injuries like hip fractures more common. Out of 25 million Americans with osteoporosis, it's estimated that 1.2 million suffer hip fractures yearly.

One large case called the Nurses Health Study looked at almost 13,000 women and vitamin K intake. The women with more vitamin K in their diet were far less likely to sustain a fractured hip by 55%. In the study, iceberg lettuce was the most common source for vitamin K, followed by broccoli, spinach, romaine lettuce, and Brussels sprouts.[13]

Another study from Japan examined 70 postmenopausal women who were experiencing reduced bone density, or weaker bones. Their blood had lower concentrations of vitamin K1 than their healthy counterparts. Several additional studies have backed up this data.

Hardening of the Arteries

Another term for this is atherosclerosis, or coronary artery disease, where the arteries harden and blood flow becomes restricted. The actual hardening process is called "vascular calcification" because the arteries are calcifying.

It appears that good vitamin K levels can prevent this, because the vitamin helps create a substance called matrix glaprotein (MGP). The more MGP you have, the less likely it is that your arteries will harden, which would lead to atherosclerosis.

Women's Health

Although not well documented, vitamin K could potentially treat heavy menstrual bleeding.

Stomach Problems

Vitamin K might be useful in offsetting nausea.

What Happens When You Don't Get Enough?

Since it is so readily obtained through diet, occasions of vitamin K deficiency are rare.

Deficiencies usually occur in those who have problems absorbing vitamins and minerals, or who have a medical condition that disrupts fat absorption. The causes include:

- Bowel obstruction
- Long-term use of antibiotics
- Ulcerative colitis
- Alcoholism
- Chronic liver disease

Supplementation may be necessary for those in this group, for newborn babies who are at risk of hemorrhaging, or for pregnant women taking anticonvulsants.

Symptoms of vitamin K deficiency include easy bruising and prolonged bleeding from minor cuts and scrapes.

Food Sources

You can get most of your vitamin K through food; and you don't need to eat a lot of vitamin-K rich foods, since it's found in such large amounts. In the case of this unusual vitamin, we're going to show here how many micrograms (mcg) these food sources have per 100 grams.

Here are the foods we can derive vitamin K from:

- Collard greens: 440 mcg/100 g
- Salad greens: 315 mcg/100 g
- Broccoli: 180 mcg/100 g
- Cabbage: 145 mcg/100 g
- Olive oil: 55 mcg/100 g
- Green beans: 33 mcg/100 g
- Spinach: 380 mcg/100 g
- Kale: 270 mcg/100 g
- Brussels sprouts: 177 mcg/100 g

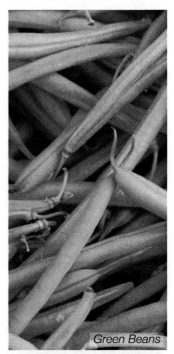
Green Beans

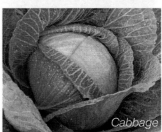
Cabbage

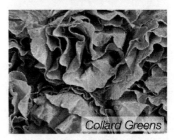
Collard Greens

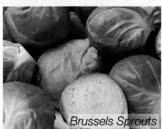
Brussels Sprouts

- Asparagus: 60 mcg/100 g
- Okra: 44 mcg/100 g
- Lentils: 22 mcg/100 g

Health Conditions

Vitamin K is useful in treating these various conditions:

- Cancer
- Low bone density
- Osteoporosis
- Hemorrhaging
- Hardening of the arteries
- Atherosclerosis
- Heavy menstrual bleeding
- Nausea

Dosage

Vitamin K is only needed in small doses, and you can get most of it from your food. Here are suggested dosages from the *U.S. Dietary Intake Reference* for people 20 and older:

Vitamin K

Recommended Daily Intake (Men):	120 mg
Recommended Daily Intake (Women):	90 mg
Maximum Recommended Intake:	Undetermined

In the studies of osteoporosis sufferers listed previously, those participants were taking vitamin K doses of approximately 110 mcg.

Possible Side Effects

Vitamin K is extremely safe, even for pregnant and breastfeeding women and/or young children. Scientists have not determined a maximum dosage amount for vitamin K.

Possible Interactions

High levels of vitamin K should not be combined with the drug warfarin. Warfarin blocks the effects from vitamin K, while vitamin K reduces the blood-thinning effects of warfarin.

Antibiotics, especially those in the group known as cephalosporins, kill the bacteria that activate vitamin K. This can cause bleeding complications for those who need the blood-clotting benefits of vitamin K.

This group of antibiotics includes:

- Cefamandole (Mandol)
- Cefoperazone (Cefobid)
- Cefmetazole (Zefazone)
- Cefotetan (Cefotan)

Women who are pregnant or breastfeeding need to supplement their vitamin K if they are taking anticonvulsants. Anticonvulsants can deplete vitamin K levels in newborns, leading to bleeding problems and abnormal facial bones.

The Latest News

New studies conducted by the Jean Mayer USDA Human Nutrition Research Center on Aging at Tufts University in Boston indicate that we are getting even less vitamin K in our diets than we thought. An additional study conducted with The Procter & Gamble Company confirmed the findings. The indication is that the current RDA for vitamin K is too small, and may not be enough to maintain good bone health. This is just another good reason for you to eat your spinach and broccoli!

Vitamin K vs. Liver Cancer

Because vitamin K promotes bone growth, researchers wanted to see if it could help women suffering viral cirrhosis avoid bone loss.

Forty women (average age: 60) were given 45 mg of vitamin K daily or a placebo. Note that this vitamin K dosage is far higher than is recommended daily.

An unexpected but happy result was that the vitamin appeared to lower the risk of liver cancer. Those receiving it were almost 90% less likely to develop liver cancer.

The researchers theorized that vitamin K could prevent malignant cells in the liver from expanding, growing, and multiplying, although more studies will be needed.

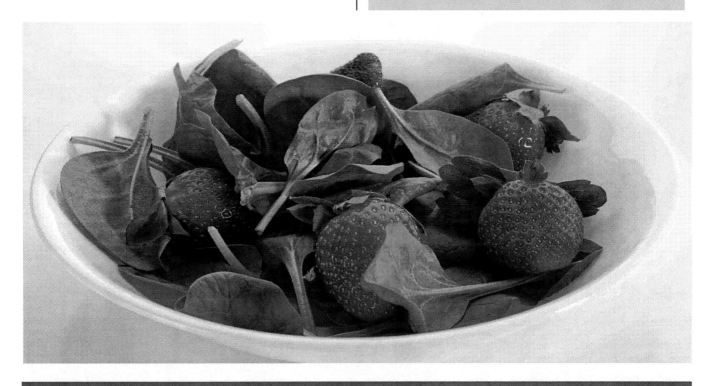

THE MINERALS

Calcium

What Is It For?

The most well-known function of calcium is in supporting healthy bones and teeth. Indeed, most of the calcium in your body is stored in your teeth, while the remaining one percent is found in the blood, muscles, and fluid between cells. Combined with vitamin D, calcium prevents osteoporosis, a bone-crippling disease. Calcium is more abundant in your body than any other mineral.

Here is what calcium has been shown effective for:

Cellular Support

A diet high in calcium has been linked with a lower risk of colon cancer. Colon cancer can develop from polyps that grow on the colon walls. Studies have shown that even people with a history of getting polyps can reduce the number of them by supplementing with calcium.

Two studies, the Nurses Healthy Study and the Physicians Health Study looked at diets and various diseases. Of the 135,000 people surveyed, those who took 700–800 mg of calcium daily cut their risk of left side colon cancer in half.[14]

Bone Health

The bone loss and hip fractures of the disease osteoporosis can be a result of low calcium intake over one's lifetime. Other factors can contribute, like a lack of vitamin D, an inability to absorb vitamin D and calcium effectively, or an excessive secretion of calcium.

Bone loss is a normal part of aging. But if you want to avoid or limit your risk of osteoporosis, you need to increase your calcium intake as time goes on. These two facts are in direct proportion to each other: more calcium = reduced risk.

Postmenopausal women can prevent this the most. In this group, supplements prevent bone loss, slow down erosion, and can even reverse the situation in some cases. Years ago, this prompted the U.S. Food & Drug Administration (FDA) to mandate special food labels reading: "Adequate calcium intake throughout life is linked to reduced risk of osteoporosis through the mechanism of optimizing peak bone mass during adolescence and early adulthood and decreasing bone loss later in life."

Some experts believe adding other trace minerals to calcium such as copper, zinc, and manganese can magnify this benefit. There have been many studies on the topic and more are in the works. What we can know for sure is that there is a definite link between calcium and osteoporosis.

High Blood Pressure

Information on whether calcium can treat this seems to go both ways. It's known that a calcium deficiency can cause hypertension. However, it's not known whether supplementing with

MINERALS 2

calcium can adjust blood pressure. Some studies seem to contradict one another.

What's known for sure is that if your diet incorporates a healthy amount of fruits, vegetables, and low-fat dairy products, this dietary intake of calcium will go a long way in controlling your blood pressure.

What Happens When You Don't Get Enough?

When you don't get enough calcium, your body steals it from your bones to ensure proper calcium levels in your blood. This is one of the reasons that calcium deficiency is so widespread and common.

In fact, up to 55% of men in North America are not getting enough calcium daily. More startling, 73% of women are not getting enough. This is why supplementation with calcium or multivitamins containing calcium is so important.

Greater risks occur for those who already suffer from a vitamin D deficiency, such as vegans, or those who do not get enough sun. Because of their diet, vegans take in far less calcium and vitamin D than others.

Low blood calcium is common with a recurring medical problem, a surgery, or the use of diuretics. In these cases, deficiency symptoms can turn fatal. You must see a doctor if you experience any of these symptoms:

- Tingling in your fingers
- Fatigue
- Mental confusion

- Muscle cramps
- Abnormal heart rhythm

Food Sources

As a kid, you were probably told to drink your milk to get healthy bones and teeth. Although that's true, there are other sources besides dairy that you can also use.

Here are the foods we can derive calcium from:

- Milk
- Cheese
- Plain yogurt
- Fruit yogurt
- Calcium-fortified orange juice
- Fortified breakfast cereal
- Tofu
- Sardines
- Salmon
- Spinach
- Kale
- Turnip greens

Health Conditions

Calcium is useful in treating these various conditions:

- Colon cancer
- Low bone density
- Osteoporosis
- High blood pressure
- Hardening of the arteries

Dosage

Calcium comes in different forms, so choosing one can be confusing. Let's look at the three supplemental options:

Natural Calcium

This form is derived naturally from bones, shells, and the earth itself. Tablets offer about 500 mg each, giving you a good-sized dose. However, some have had concerns over the levels of lead in these tablets and whether this makes them unsafe, since amounts are not indicated on labels.

Calcium Carbonate

This is the one you see on drugstore shelves most often. It has a low cost, but many people have trouble absorbing it, especially those who have low stomach acid levels. So for this form, it's recommended that you take it with your food. The process that will have already started to break down your food will handle the calcium tablet too, and make it easier for your body to absorb.

Chelated Calcium

In this form, the calcium is bound to an organic acid. It's designed to make the calcium more absorbable than calcium carbonate. Usually the acid used is a form of citric acid, or citrates. Two of them, calcium citrate and calcium citrate malate, are commonly prescribed by doctors. The down side is that this form is more expensive and bulkier. To get the desired benefits, you may have to take five big pills daily.

Calcium

Recommended Daily Intake (Men):	1,000 mg
Recommended Daily Intake (Women):	1,000 mg
Recommended Daily Intake (Men over 50):	1,200 mg
Recommended Daily Intake (Women over 50):	1,200 mg
Maximum Recommended Intake:	Undetermined

Since your body can only absorb 500 mg of calcium at any given time, these dosages need to be broken up and taken throughout the day.

If you're aiming to prevent bone loss, supplement with calcium regularly and for the long term; once you stop, the improvements disappear quickly.

Possible Side Effects

Calcium is very safe to take, even in large doses. However, excessively high doses can produce calcium deposits in your body that can lead

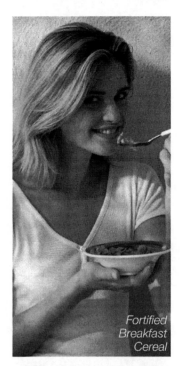

Fortified Breakfast Cereal

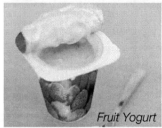

Fruit Yogurt

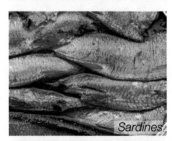

Sardines

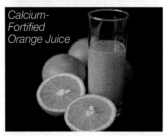

Calcium-Fortified Orange Juice

MINERALS 2

to painful conditions, such as kidney stones.

Side effects are minor, including:

- Bloating
- Gas
- Constipation

Possible Interactions

If you have any of the following conditions, do not take calcium without first consulting your doctor:

- Kidney stones
- Kidney disease
- Thyroid-related disorders
- Sarcoidosis
- Prostate cancer

Use caution if taking any of the following medications, because supplementing with calcium may hinder the absorption of the drug or the mineral itself:

- Calcium channel blockers
- Antibiotics (tetracycline, fluoroquinolone)
- Corticosteroids
- Antacids containing aluminum

- Beta-blockers
- Thiazide diuretics
- Anticonvulsants
- Levothyroxine

If your doctor has approved your use of calcium in these situations, be sure to take your calcium supplement more than two hours before or after taking any medication.

Calcium may interfere with your body's absorption of magnesium, iron, zinc, and manganese.

The Latest News

There may be a link between calcium and ovarian cancer. A recent study from the Wake Forest Baptist Medical Center is the first one reporting the prediction of ovarian cancers by examining blood calcium levels. The study found that calcium blood levels were higher in those with ovarian cancer who eventually became fatalities. High calcium is connected with rare forms of ovarian cancer, and researchers want to determine if other forms of cancer could be connected to lower calcium blood levels. The research is still ongoing.

Chromium

What Is It For?

Here is what chromium has been shown effective for:

Blood Sugar

Chromium is important to the regulation of blood sugar (glucose), working hand-in-hand with another better-known component, insulin. Our bodies use insulin to regulate the movement of glucose in and out of cells. Meanwhile, chromium keeps blood sugar amounts at a functional level and helps the body use it correctly.

For these reasons, chromium supplements may be beneficial to diabetics. Studies have shown that large doses of chromium can help type 2 diabetes patients control their glucose. It also allowed them to cut back on oral medications and insulin they had been taking.

Chromium has been particularly helpful to pregnant women who also develop diabetes.

On the other side of the coin, chromium can benefit those with glucose intolerance and insulin resistance by supplementing with this mineral. This is because chromium improves your body's response to insulin.

Weight Loss

Although various studies have been done on the impact chromium can have on weight loss, there is no definitive answer yet, and results have appeared mixed. Athletes and body builders swear by chromium for fat burning and lean muscle mass.

A significant study involved 150 people in a double-blind trial. They were given two different chromium doses or a placebo for over three months. The group taking chromium experienced a loss of fat and leaner body mass, accompanied by measurable weight loss. The placebo group gained none of these benefits.[15]

While this was a very large and encouraging study, other smaller studies seem to contradict the results.

High Cholesterol

Clinically known as hyperlipidemia, this condition accelerates the risk of heart disease. Chromium can improve cholesterol levels in the bloodstream, as it reduces LDL levels, and raises HDL levels. This gives you a better lipid profile, a test used to determine one's risk of heart disease. These improvements have been seen with doses of 250 micrograms daily.

Combined with exercise, the improvements can be even more pronounced. By the way, this is true for all the vitamins and minerals in this book. You should always try to add exercise with your supplementation for overall health and vitamin effectiveness.

Headaches

It's been suggested that chromium can be of great benefit to migraine sufferers, but as of today, there is still not a lot of hard evidence.

Skin Problems

Likewise, chromium has been used for skin conditions such as acne and psoriasis, but there is no overwhelming evidence to suggest a link.

What Happens When You Don't Get Enough?

Deficiencies in chromium are difficult to measure in any reliable way. However, it is known that most of us do not get the recommended amounts of this mineral each day.

Doctors are recommending more chromium supplementation due to the rise in diabetes, obesity, and poor diets, due to chromium's regulating power over blood sugar.

A lack of chromium could very well lead to diabetes and the inability for the body to use sugar properly.

Chromium deficiency may also contribute to the following conditions:

- Weight loss
- Neurological disorders (numbness or tingling in the extremities)
- Reduced resistance to infection
- Sexual dysfunction
- Cataracts

Food Sources

The database on chromium and its amounts in food is thin, at best. However, the following are believed to be the richest sources of chromium:

- Broccoli
- Whole grains
- Potatoes
- Tomatoes
- Liver
- Green beans
- Romaine lettuce
- Nuts
- Brewer's yeast
- Grape juice
- Onions (raw)
- Fresh fruit and vegetables

Health Conditions

Chromium can be useful in treating these various conditions:

- Glucose intolerance
- Insulin resistance
- Diabetes
- Obesity
- Weight loss
- High cholesterol
- Migraine headaches
- Acne
- Psoriasis

Dosage

Most daily doses are safe, but if you are going to supplement to levels of 1,000 mcg, you should first consult your doctor.

If you are trying to regulate your blood sugar levels or ward off diabetes, you should take the form of this mineral called chromium piccolinate. This has been shown to have the best results. Long-term use of this supplement has been problematic for some, so it's recommended that you consult your doctor before supplementing with it.

Chromium

Recommended Daily Intake (Men):	50-300 mcg
Recommended Daily Intake (Women):	50-300 mcg
Maximum Recommended Intake:	1,000 mcg

Possible Side Effects

Chromium has not been linked to any toxicity, and the recommended dosages are perfectly safe.

While some people have experienced problems dosing in the 200–400-microgram range, the toxicity may have been linked to the presence of hepatic or renal disease. This group experienced impaired memory, motor, and sensory functions, and eventually kidney or liver problems. Keep in mind that these are a handful of cases, again, where disease may already have been present.

There are theories that chromium can be altered by antioxidants, leading to damage from free radicals and increased cancer risk, but there is no current solid evidence for this.

Warnings About Interactions

Not much is known about possible drug interactions with chromium. However, one positive interaction may be chromium's ability to return HDL cholesterol levels to normal in those who take beta-blockers. The beta-blockers disrupt healthy lipid levels, but the chromium can offset this problem.

Two minerals, when taken in high doses, are thought to decrease your body's absorption of chromium: calcium and magnesium.

Conversely, non-steroidal anti-inflammatories (NSAIDs) can increase your chromium absorption and retention, resulting in higher blood levels of chromium.

These drugs may also affect your chromium levels:

- Antacids
- Corticosteroids
- H2-blockers
- Proton pump inhibitors

The Latest News

An overlooked form of chromium may be the answer to wiping out diabetes. It's called whole foods grown GTF chromium, and it's being theorized that 100 mcg taken three times daily along with modest regular physical activity and a reasonably healthy diet could not only eliminate diabetes, but could save our health care system $100 billion annually. GTF chromium may have been kept quiet because the government actually owns the patent on chromium piccolinate.

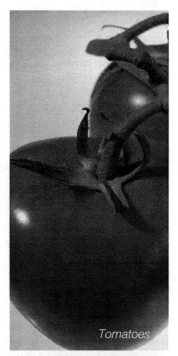

Tomatoes

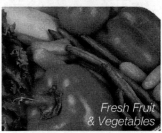

Fresh Fruit & Vegetables

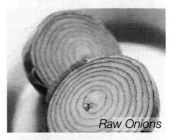

Raw Onions

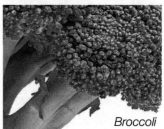

Broccoli

MINERALS 2

Copper

What Is It For?

Copper is a trace mineral that generally supports your body's processes and enhances other vitamins and minerals. It's more of a "behind the scenes" player rather than a definitive disease fighter. Your body needs it, but generally, you don't take it to target a specific disease. You take it to promote general health and bodily function.

There are plenty of amateur theories about diseases that copper can treat, but most are not backed up by any specific scientific evidence. They claim that copper can decrease your risk for heart disease, lower your cholesterol, and treat arthritis. Be careful of claims that seem too good to be true.

Bone Health

This is an area that has been looked at closely, because the common theory has been that copper can treat osteoporosis. Again, there isn't any proven evidence that it does so by itself, but it may have a beneficial result when combined with several other minerals.

One reliable study was done looking at copper's possible link to bone formation. In the study, 16 young women were given high doses of copper in the 3–6-gram range, over month-long periods. It was found that the copper supplements had no effect on the building of bone.

What Happens When You Don't Get Enough?

Although copper deficiencies are uncommon in North America, it's also still true that most people don't get enough. We should all be taking in 1.5–3 mg daily, which is a healthy dosage range.

There are certain groups who are more at risk for copper deficiency. They include the following:

- Premature infants
- Babies fed only milk past their first year
- People with severe intestinal disorders (this affects copper absorption)

The symptoms of copper deficiency are:
- Anemia
- Heart defects
- Infertility
- Hair loss
- Nerve damage
- Skeletal deformation

Food Sources

Yes, you can actually get copper through your diet. It's abundant in some foods.

Here are the foods we can derive copper from:
- Oysters (raw)
- Wheat bran, wheat germ

- Shellfish
- Turnip greens
- Kale
- Green olives
- Legumes (dried beans and peas)
- Organ meats
- Crimini mushrooms
- Avocados
- Brazil nuts, other nuts and seeds

Health Conditions

Although it is just theory with no real hard evidence to back it up, it's believed that copper can be useful in treating these various conditions:

- Osteoporosis
- Heart disease
- High cholesterol
- Arthritis

Dosage

Most doctors support supplementing with copper, since so few of us actually get enough in our diet.

Other supplements can affect the absorption of copper in your body. Therefore, if you take any of these, it's recommended that you supplement with copper as well:

- Zinc
- Vitamin C
- Manganese

These certain medical conditions also affect your body's absorption of copper:

- Chronic diarrhea
- Celiac disease
- Crohn's disease

Copper

Recommended Daily Intake (Men):	1-3 mcg
Recommended Daily Intake (Women):	1-3 mcg
Maximum Recommended Intake:	10 mcg

If you get your drinking water from copper pipes, you may already be getting your daily requirements.

Consult your doctor before supplementing with copper. Kidney failure and death can occur with ingesting as little as one gram of copper sulfate.

Possible Side Effects

Copper is safe at the nutritional levels listed. The upper levels that could cause you problems is not exactly known, but some have reported nausea at doses of 10 mg and vomiting at doses of 60 mg.

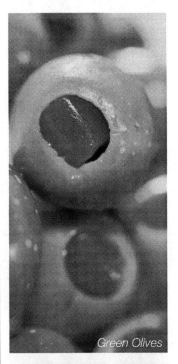

Green Olives

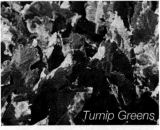

Turnip Greens

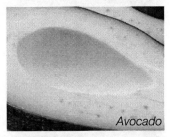

Avocado

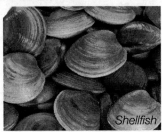

Shellfish

If you're taking zinc, copper is safe up to three milligrams daily.

Warnings About Interactions

Along with zinc, vitamin C, and manganese, antacids can limit your body's absorption of copper. This is because antacids limit the available stomach acid needed to process it.

On the other hand, birth control pills actually increase the body's absorption of copper.

As far as drug interactions, the copper level in your blood may be reduced when taking AZT.

Conversely, copper might enhance the effects of non-steroidal anti-inflammatories (NSAIDs):

- Ibuprofen
- Naproxen
- Oxaprozin
- Etodolac

The Latest News

Researchers in The Birchall Centre at Keele University, Staffordshire, U.K. have discovered that copper can protect against Alzheimer's disease. Deposits known as senile plaques result from certain protein buildups, which then damage the brain. This usually results when there are low levels of copper in the brain. It was once thought that copper actually caused the plaques or contributed to their formation somehow, but more recent research suggests the opposite seems to be true.

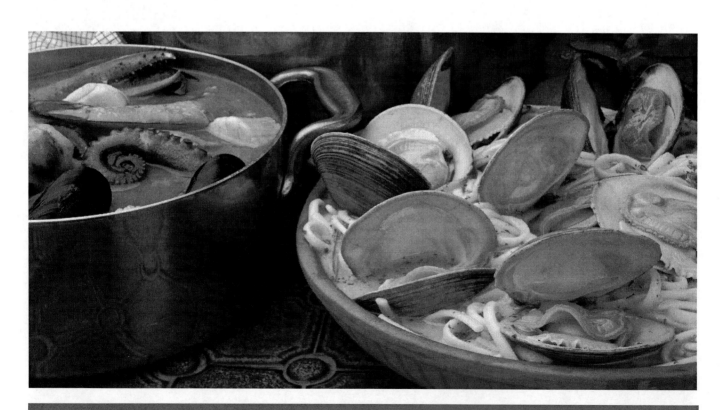

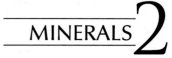

Iodine

What Is It For?

The main function of iodine in your body is in the creation of vital hormones. It's one link in a chain of events that happens when your hormone levels drop.

First, the pituitary gland recognizes the drop in hormones. It then sends a message to your thyroid with tiny messengers we'll call thyroid-stimulating hormones. The thyroid obeys the messages by taking more iodine from your bloodstream. Finally, once it has this extra material, it begins to manufacture the missing hormones, thereby bringing your levels back up to where they should be.

Here is what iodine is believed to be effective for:

Germ Fighting

For many years, iodine capsules have been used to purify water for campers, military personnel, and others. This is because iodine kills harmful bacteria. Iodine capsules can be easily added to canteens or containers, making the water from lakes and streams safe to drink.

These same qualities are why iodine has been used topically as a skin disinfectant in homes and hospitals. Iodine is also an effective antiseptic.

Immune System

It's thought that a deficiency in iodine can impair your immune system.

Cellular Health

Iodine can improve the symptoms of a thyroid condition. It also promotes hormone creation.

Respiratory Problems

Taken orally, iodine acts as an expectorant to help clear up respiratory congestion.

Women's Health

Iodine may play an important role in women's breast health.

Often associated with premenstrual syndrome, there is a condition called cyclic mastalgia, also known as fibrocystic breast disease. It makes the breast unusually lumpy and tender, sometimes accompanied by pain and a dull heaviness. When the lumps grow, they can trick mammograms into falsely indicating the presence of breast cancer.

Some studies suggest that iodine can relieve the pain and reduce the number of cysts resulting from this disease.

What Happens When You Don't Get Enough?

Iodine deficiency used to be common until the 20th century, when iodized salt was introduced. The resulting benefit was then given to animals in their feed, which has resulted in an iodine infusion in many of the products we buy at the grocery store, including milk.

Some countries still experience iodine deficiencies, due to shunning iodized salt in favor of natural salt.

MINERALS 2

The main result of an iodine deficiency is goiter. Goiter results when the pituitary gland sends too many of its hormone messengers to your thyroid, basically over stimulating it. The thyroid will then try unsuccessfully to manufacture more hormones without the iodine it needs to do so.

The symptoms of iodine deficiency match those of an underactive thyroid. They include:

- Dry skin
- Sudden weight gain
- Fatigue
- Slow reflexes
- Difficulty concentrating
- Raised cholesterol levels

If eaten in large amounts, certain foods can actually block your body's absorption of iodine. They include:

- Cruciferous vegetables (broccoli, cauliflower)
- Soy
- Mustard
- Millet

Overconsumption of these can lead to thyroid problems, unless they are cooked.

Food Sources

Iodine is abundant in many foods. Here are some we can derive iodine from:

- Iodized salt
- Seafood (especially shellfish)
- Milk
- Strawberries
- Sea vegetables (kelp, seaweed)
- Low-fat yogurt
- Eggs

Health Conditions

It's believed that iodine can be useful in treating these various conditions:

- Low hormones
- Bacterial infection
- Impaired immune system
- Thyroid conditions
- Respiratory congestion
- Fibrocystic breast disease

Dosage

Elemental iodine is found in supplements as caseinate and within products that contain kelp. Many supplements blend iodine with potassium or sodium.

Iodine

Recommended Daily Intake (Men):	150 mcg
Recommended Daily Intake (Women):	150 mcg
Pregnant or Nursing Women:	180-200 mcg
Maximum Recommended Intake:	1,1000 mcg

Possible Side Effects

Iodine as a supplement is reasonably safe. One need not have concern unless it's being taken in high doses, because this could actually have the opposite effect of impairing your thyroid, rather than supporting it.

It would be very difficult to overdose on iodine through dietary sources. The most a man could end up getting would be perhaps 300 micrograms in one day; for a woman, 210 micrograms. Even getting slightly more than recommended levels are tolerated by the body just fine.

Overusing iodine will show up as the following symptoms:

- Sore gums and teeth
- Burning in the mouth
- Increased saliva
- Eye irritation
- Headache
- Coughing
- Swelling
- Skin lesions
- Diarrhea
- Depression
- Stomach upset

At a high level of one gram or more, symptoms will become more serious. These will include:

- Burning sensation in the mouth
- Burning sensation in the throat
- Burning sensation in the stomach
- Abdominal pain
- Nausea
- Vomiting
- Diarrhea

Finally, if your body cannot dispel such a large amount, there is a possibility that you could become comatose. This is a phenomenally rare occurrence, but it does happen.

Warnings About Interactions

Do not take any thyroid medications while taking iodine without first consulting your doctor.

Combining iodine with angiotensin receptor blockers or ACE inhibitors increases the risk of hyperkalemia, or dangerously high potassium levels.

Some chemicals contain high levels of iodine, and can have an impact on your thyroid. These include amiodarone, a heart medication, and erythrosine, a red food coloring.

Obviously, you would not want to be supplementing with iodine if you are taking either of these.

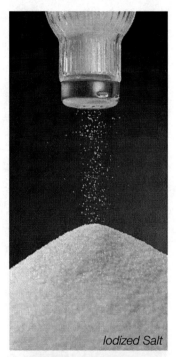

Iodized Salt

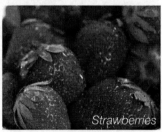

Strawberries

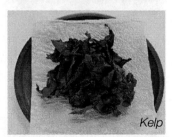

Kelp

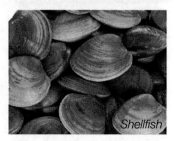

Shellfish

MINERALS 2

The Latest News

Iodine deficiency in pregnant women appears to be tied to a number of negative health consequences, including low IQ in the baby, according to a professor of obstetrics and gynecology at the George Washington University (GW) School of Medicine and Health Sciences. Iodine deficiency is the leading cause of preventable mental retardation globally. Other risks include maternal and fetal goiter, increased pregnancy loss, and infant death.

Organizations like the American Thyroid Association recommend iodine supplementation for pregnant and lactating mothers, but most prenatal vitamins on the market don't contain iodine. Studies have shown that only 20% of women in the U.S. are taking iodine supplements. Researchers recommend 150 mcg of potassium iodide daily for pregnant women.

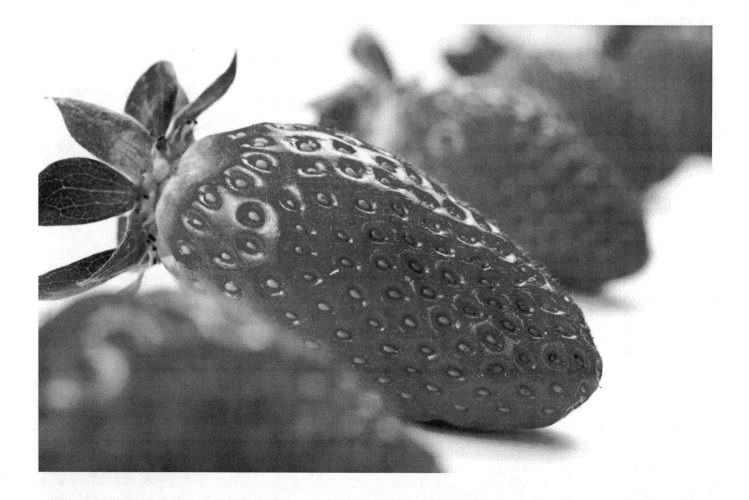

Iron

What Is It For?

Here is what iron is believed to be effective for:

Better Exercise

Whether you're a professional athlete or average person, iron may give you the benefits of a better workout, especially when it comes to aerobic fitness.

One study looked at 42 women who were known to have lower iron levels. Taking iron supplements increased the benefits of their workouts, giving them much bigger gains in speed and endurance compared to others in the group who were given a placebo.[16]

Immune System

Many cases have found that AIDS and HIV-positive patients are deficient in iron. Supplementation with iron could benefit them.

Restless Legs Syndrome

Although the evidence is weak, iron may play a role in alleviating the inner "crawling" sensations of restless legs syndrome. Some subjects given iron supplements appeared to have reduced symptoms. However, if you already have adequate iron levels in your body, supplements will not help.

Attention Deficit Disorder (ADD)

Again, here the evidence is scant, but iron has been used as a treatment for ADD.

Women's Health

Decades ago, research showed that iron supplements could help women suffering menorrhagia, or heavy menstruation. Three quarters of women studied saw improvements in their condition.

However, women who entered the study with high levels of iron saw no real benefit. The conclusion has been that people should supplement with iron only if they are among those who are deficient.

Brain Health

Iron has been shown to improve the cognitive function of children who have an iron deficiency.

What Happens When You Don't Get Enough?

Iron is the number one mineral deficiency in the world, according to the World Health Organization (WHO). As many as 80% of people across the globe have inadequate amounts. Worse, about 30% of the population may have anemia due to lack of iron.

Anemia occurs when you have a large drop in the number of red blood cells. Anemia produces the following symptoms:

- Paleness
- Fatigue
- Shortness of breath
- Rapid heartbeat
- Dizziness
- Cold hands
- Higher risk of infection

MINERALS 2

Even without the presence of anemia, iron deficiency still can show symptoms. They include:

- Feeling tired
- Feeling weak
- Poor performance at work or school
- Slow childhood social and mental development
- Fluctuating body temperature
- Depressed immune system
- Inflamed tongue

This results from not enough oxygen getting to your cells. Another weird symptom of iron deficiency can cause you to develop cravings for certain foods, or in severe cases, non-food items.

There are at-risk groups who need more iron as a natural result of their situation or lifestyle. These are people who need to supplement to supply what their body needs:

- Pregnant women (the growth of the child means they need three-times more iron than a man)
- Menstruating women (because of blood loss)
- Vegetarians (iron isn't absorbed as well through vegetables)
- Children and teens (still growing and developing)
- Dieters
- Frequent blood donors (iron is necessary to rebuild the blood)
- Kidney failure patients

Food Sources

There are two forms of dietary iron: heme and non-heme. Heme iron comes from hemoglobin and myoglobin. It's found in animal foods containing these blood cells, namely, red meat, fish, and poultry.

Non-heme is where you get the bulk of your dietary iron, and it's found in plants. However, it's not absorbed as well as heme iron. Overall, your body absorbs about 10%–15% of the iron in your food.

Here are the foods we can derive heme iron from:

- Red meat
- Poultry
- Oysters and other shellfish
- Fish

Here are the dietary sources of non-heme iron:

- Whole grains
- Dried fruits (apricots, raisins)
- Kelp
- Seeds
- Legumes (especially soybeans)
- Dark green leafy vegetables
- Egg yolks
- Fortified cereals and breads

Believe it or not, the type of cookware you use can influence your iron intake! When you cook foods with high acidity like tomatoes or fruit preserves in iron or stainless steel pans, some of the mineral will actually become part of your food.

Health Conditions

It's believed that iron can be useful in treating these various conditions:

- Poor aerobic fitness levels
- Impaired immune system
- Restless legs syndrome
- Attention deficit disorder
- Heavy menstruation
- Anemia
- Cognitive function
- Pica
- Food pica

Dosage

Not all iron supplements are equal, and it's important to know the differences based on your needs.

Ferrous iron is more easily absorbed than ferric iron. Ferrous sulfate is most commonly used in supplements. However, these pills may be enteric-coated to prevent any side effects once in your intestinal system. This coating can make the iron less absorbable.

The best ones to look for will have these names:

- Ferrous fumarate
- Ferrous gluconate
- Heme iron concentrate
- Iron glycine amino acid chelate

These versions are easily absorbed and cause fewer side effects. NOTE: Always take your iron with food.

Also, doctors do not recommend iron supplements for men or expecting mothers unless they have an iron deficiency. A blood test should be performed first to check iron blood levels.

Here are suggested dosages for specific groups:

Iron

Recommended Daily Intake (Men):	8 mg
Recommended Daily Intake (Women):	18 mg
Recommended Daily Intake (Men over 50):	8 mg
Recommended Daily Intake (Women over 50):	8 mg
Pregnant Women	27-45 mg
Vegetarians/Vegans	33 mg
Maximum Recommended Intake (short-term only):	100-200 mg

Possible Side Effects

Excessive iron levels can provoke too many oxidants in your blood and may restrict blood

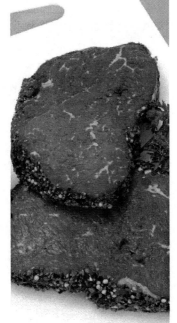

Red Meat

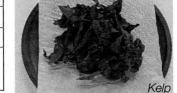

Chicken

Kelp

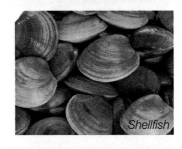

Shellfish

flow. This could also starve your cells of much-needed oxygen. The oxidation could lead to:

- Increased risk of heart disease
- Increased risk of cancer
- Neuronal injury
- Pregnancy complications

Adverse reactions at doses below 45 mg are uncommon. Some may experience more minor issues when taking iron supplements, such as:

- Cramping
- Bloating
- Constipation
- Nausea

Possible Interactions

Taking the following with your supplements could reduce your body's absorption of iron:

- Coffee
- Tea
- Dairy products

Conversely, taking high doses of vitamin C with iron will cause excessive iron absorption.

When taking iron and zinc together, make sure you eat first; otherwise, the two will inhibit the absorption of each other.

Likewise, the same effect can happen when taking iron with certain medications and chemicals. These include:

- Antibiotics (quinolone, tetracycline families)
- Methyldopa

- Levodopa
- Carbidopa
- Penicillamine
- Thyroid hormone
- ACE inhibitors
- H-2 blockers
- Calcium, zinc, copper, or manganese
- Antacids

A Little Bird Told Us

A strange medical condition called pica can result from an iron deficiency. It's named after a bird that eats almost anything.

Pica sufferers have been known to crave dirt, chalk, paper, paint chips, cardboard, "Styrofoam," rust, cigarette butts, paste, ice chips, and more. In one case, a woman ate her own socks!

Pica can be influenced by social or psychological factors, too. In the case of the woman and her socks, she had anxiety about moving away from home in addition to her iron deficiency.

A less abstract version of pica exists called food pica. It's more common in North America, and finds the iron-deficient person compulsively chewing ice, salty potato chips, pickles, and under-ripe fruit. In all cases, iron supplements can halt this strange eating disorder.

- Chloramphenicol
- Proton pump inhibitors
- Soy

The Latest News

A recent study found that giving iron supplements to infants with a low birthweight will reduce the risk of ADHD later in life. Researchers in Sweden did a randomized controlled trial with 285 low birthweight infants. They received no iron, 1 mg/kg of iron, or 2 mg/kg of iron daily from the ages of six weeks to six months. At age three and a half, the children were assessed for behavior and intelligence. There were 95 children of normal birthweight who were also tested.

When tested for behavioral problems, iron seemed to have an impact. Of those who took no iron, 12.7% showed signs of ADHD. In the one-mg/kg group, 2.9% showed signs of ADHD, while a lower 2.7% of those in the two-mg/kg group showed signs of ADHD.

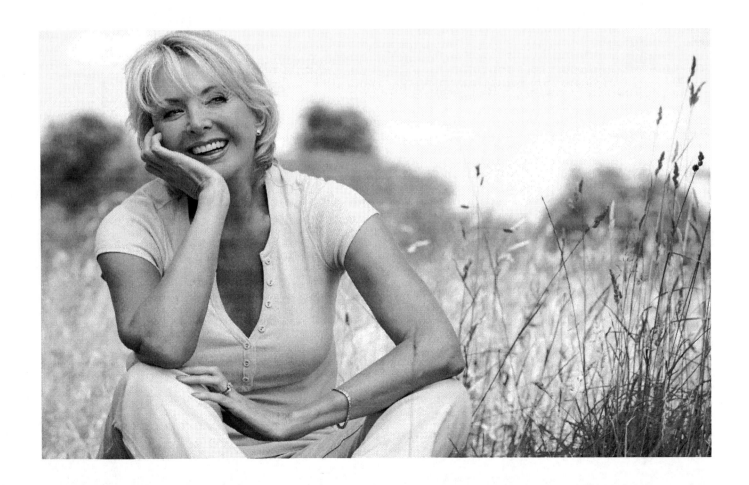

MINERALS 2

Magnesium

What Is It For?

Here is what magnesium is believed to be effective for:

Hearing Loss

Even in small amounts, magnesium has been found to help prevent hearing loss. This is a boon to those who work around extremely loud noises and environments.

In one two-month study, researchers gave 300 military recruits magnesium supplements of 167 mg daily. Although this is way below the recommended daily intake, the soldiers still experienced beneficial results: both the incidence and severity of hearing loss from high-volume noise was reduced.[17]

Heart Health

Magnesium supplements can help the dangerous condition known as coronary artery disease.

High doses of magnesium at 1,000 mg daily, may improve the tolerance for exercise in those with heart disease.

Low levels of magnesium in the body may cause irregular heart rhythms and unwanted metabolic changes that lead to heart problems.

Intravenous doses of magnesium can actually correct many types of irregular heart rhythms.

Headaches

There's a lot of evidence proving magnesium's effectiveness against migraine headaches. In one study, 80 patients were given 600 mg of magnesium daily or a placebo for a period of three months. The magnesium significantly reduced the frequency of their migraines by over 40%. Others have backed up this study.[18]

Women's Health

Magnesium can improve a painful, menstruation-related condition known as dysmenorrhea. The theory is that this mineral depletes the amount of a particular prostaglandin that contributes to dysmenorrhea.

The symptoms of PMS can also be positively impacted by magnesium supplements. These include:

- Mood swings
- Fluid retention
- Headaches

Kidney Stones

The calcium-blocking effects of magnesium may be able to halt the growth of painful kidney stones. While this has not been definitively proven as yet, there have been very promising test results. At the very least, getting your magnesium every day can reduce the risk of kidney stones.

High Blood Pressure

Studies have showed conflicting results as to whether magnesium alone can lower blood pressure. However, what is known for sure is that people with healthy diets who are getting magnesium and potassium are less prone to high blood pressure. It may be that the combination of the two is what has the effect.

Children's Autism

Six studies carried out by one research group

have shown that combining magnesium with vitamin B6 produces improvements in autistic behavior.

Other Conditions

Magnesium is a mineral that has wide-ranging effects throughout your body. This may be why there are many medical claims that magnesium can help with numerous conditions, including:

- Constipation
- Osteoporosis
- Fibromyalgia
- Preeclampsia
- Diabetes
- Attention deficit disorder
- Alzheimer's disease
- Periodontal disease
- Restless legs syndrome
- Arthritis

What Happens When You Don't Get Enough?

Magnesium deficiency is common in North America. This can be dietary, or you may be losing too much through urination. You may have a gastrointestinal system that has trouble absorbing magnesium, or a low intake of the mineral for extended periods. Vomiting and diarrhea can deplete your magnesium reserves.

Those who suffer from low calcium or potassium levels may have an underlying magnesium deficiency.

Severe magnesium deficiency can be brought on by the following medical conditions:

- Kidney disease
- Alcoholism
- Malabsorption disorders
- Hyperparathyroidism

The symptoms of severe magnesium deficiency include:

- Confusion
- Disorientation
- Loss of appetite
- Depression
- Painful muscle cramps
- Tingling and numbness
- Seizures
- Abnormal heart rhythms
- Fatigue
- Listlessness
- Personality changes

Before attempting to improve any of these conditions with supplements, you should consult your doctor, because some people are at a higher risk of deficiency than others.

Food Sources

Like any other nutrient, there is far less magnesium in refined food than in whole foods. For instance, white bread has only half the magnesium of whole wheat bread. This is because the process that creates refined flours also kills the nutrients.

Here are some good dietary sources of magnesium:

- Kelp
- Whole grains

MINERALS 2

- Wheat bran/germ
- Nuts (almonds and cashews)
- Brewer's yeast
- Legumes
- Avocados
- Fortified cereal
- Pumpkin seeds
- Spinach
- Collard or dandelion greens
- Sweet corn
- Cheddar cheese
- Sunflower seeds
- Soybeans
- Lentils
- Shrimp
- Peanut butter
- Antacids and laxatives containing magnesium

Health Conditions

It's believed that magnesium can be useful in treating these various conditions:

- Hearing loss
- Coronary artery disease
- Heart disease
- Irregular heart rhythms
- Migraines
- Dysmenorrhea
- PMS
- Kidney stones
- Children's autism
- Constipation
- Osteoporosis
- Fibromyalgia
- Preeclampsia
- Diabetes
- Attention deficit disorder
- Alzheimer's disease
- Periodontal disease
- Restless legs syndrome
- Arthritis

Dosage

It's safe to take magnesium supplements, even if you don't have the symptoms of deficiency. This is because our diets are so low in magnesium. Many doctors advise their patients to take 350 mg daily.

Since magnesium can interfere with other minerals, the best form will probably be found in a multi-mineral supplement rather than by itself.

Here are suggested dosages for specific groups:

Magnesium

Recommended Daily Intake (Men):	350 mg
Recommended Daily Intake (Women):	250 mg
Recommended Daily Intake (Men over 30):	420 mg
Recommended Daily Intake (Women over 30):	320 mg
Women with Menstrual Problems	500-1,000 mg*
Migraine Sufferers	600-1,800 mg
Maximum Recommended Intake:	600 mg

*This supplementation should begin on day 15 of your cycle.

Consult your doctor before taking large doses.

Possible Side Effects

In regular doses, magnesium is very safe to take.

Excessive doses of magnesium can cause the following:

- Gastrointestinal irritation
- Nausea
- Diarrhea
- Vomiting

People who suffer with kidney or heart disease should NEVER take magnesium, unless recommended by a doctor.

Magnesium can disrupt certain medications and leave you more prone to the symptoms you were medicating to prevent.

Possible Interactions

If you take the following, you should make sure you are taking extra magnesium:

- Calcium
- Zinc
- Manganese
- Oral contraceptives

Oral contraceptives cause your body to draw more of your magnesium into the bones and body tissues, thereby lowering your overall levels.

Certain drugs may lead to magnesium depletion or poorer absorption. These include:

- Diuretics
- ACE inhibitors
- H-2 blockers
- Dilantin
- Macrodantin
- Antibiotics
- Bisphosphonates
- Calcium channel blockers
- Aminoglycosides
- Cholestyramine
- Corticosteroids
- Cyclosporine
- Digoxin
- Loop diuretics

The Latest News

New discoveries show that magnesium has powerful benefits in reducing inflammation. These were found quite by chance in pregnancy studies, as magnesium sulfate is given to many women to treat preeclampsia and preterm labor. Magnesium reduces the body's production of cytokines, molecules that cause inflammation. Researchers from Case Western Reserve University School of Medicine found the mechanism by which magnesium does this, which may be a significant breakthrough in treating respiratory distress syndrome, asthma, atherosclerosis, cancer, diabetes, and other conditions marked by inflammation. Magnesium can also prevent cerebral palsy.

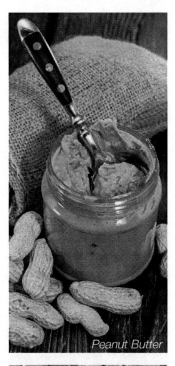

Peanut Butter

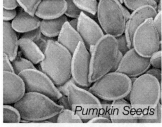

Pumpkin Seeds

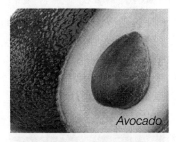

Avocado

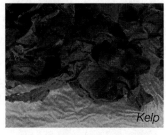

Kelp

Manganese

What Is It For?

Manganese is a form of metal. It's a part of plant and animal tissue.

In our bodies, manganese is a part of many integral enzymes in small amounts. It resides in our liver, kidney, pancreas, and bones.

Here is what manganese is believed to be effective for:

Cellular Support

Manganese is one part of an important antioxidant in your body, an enzyme known as superoxide dismutase (SOD). Manganese takes part in finding free radicals, neutralizing them and preventing the extensive damage they can cause, including cancer.

Manganese is a part of the enzymes that form connective tissue and bones, control sex hormones, synthesize cholesterol and DNA, and promote blood clotting (together with vitamin K).

Your thyroid function is influenced by manganese as well. It also contributes to the growth of healthy skin.

Bone Health

Conditions involving your bones and the benefits of manganese have the strongest available evidence. It's necessary for good, healthy bones, and may be a candidate for treating osteoporosis too.

Its best results are seen when combined with other elements such as calcium, zinc, and copper. Measurable increases of bone density in patients have occurred, especially in women.

Blood Sugar

Manganese helps control your blood sugar and glucose tolerance.

Energy and Metabolism

The metabolism of fats and carbohydrates gets an assist from this metal.

Women's Health

It's believed that when used as part of a multimineral supplement, manganese can help with menstrual pain and PMS.

Nervous System

The function of your nerves is enhanced by manganese.

Brain Health

Manganese supports your brain functions.

Other Conditions

Although the evidence is weak, there are medical claims that manganese can help with other conditions including:

- Tardive dyskinesia
- Rheumatoid Arthritis
- Diabetes

What Happens When You Don't Get Enough?

A deficiency in manganese is quite rare, because this mineral is found in a wide spectrum of foods. Of course, it's important to consume whole grains and not processed or refined grains. This along with other dietary sources will keep your manganese levels up.

There are certain groups who are more prone to experiencing manganese deficiencies. They occur in those with the following medical conditions:

- Children with birth defects
- Multiple sclerosis
- Epilepsy
- Lou Gehrig's disease

The symptoms of severe manganese deficiency include:

- Skin problems
- Difficulty in blood clotting
- Changes to the hue of hair color
- Lowered cholesterol levels
- Infertility
- Malformed bones
- Weakness
- Seizures

Food Sources

Here are some good dietary sources of manganese:

- Pineapple
- Potatoes
- Romaine lettuce
- Mustard greens
- Spinach
- Collard greens
- Turnip greens
- Garlic
- Tofu (soybeans)
- Kale
- Chard
- Legumes (green peas, beans)
- Asparagus
- Beets
- Grapes
- Raspberries
- Nuts and seeds
- Whole grains (especially oats and wheat)

And also in the following spices:

- Turmeric
- Cinnamon
- Cloves
- Thyme
- Black pepper

Health Conditions

It's believed that manganese can be useful in treating these various conditions:

- Low antioxidant levels
- Poor enzymes
- Low thyroid function
- Poor bone health
- Osteoporosis
- Weak tissue and bones
- Poor blood clotting

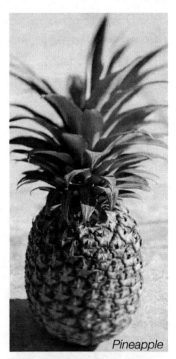

Pineapple

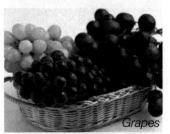

Potatoes

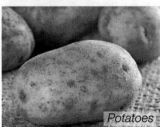

Grapes

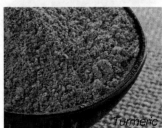

Turmeric

MINERALS 2

- Low sex hormones
- Cholesterol levels
- Skin problems
- Blood sugar
- Glucose tolerance
- Low metabolism
- Menstrual pain
- PMS
- Nerve damage
- Poor brain function
- Tardive dyskinesia
- Rheumatoid Arthritis
- Diabetes

Dosage

Although the dosages you need are small, there have been studies done using much more. These were done to see if manganese could help heal muscle sprains or strains. Those patients received anywhere from 50 mg to 200 mg daily for a two-week period following the injury.

Here are regular suggested dosages:

Manganese

Recommended Daily Intake (Men):	2.3-5 mg
Recommended Daily Intake (Women):	1.8-5 mg
Maximum Recommended Intake:	6-11 mg

Possible Side Effects

In regular doses, manganese is very safe to take. When you go above 11 mg, the safety for this mineral isn't exactly known. The symptoms of toxicity for manganese are absent when it's taken orally. However, those who have inhaled manganese vapors, like mine or mill workers, have experienced adverse effects, including:

- Headaches
- Rigid muscles
- Irritability
- Convulsions
- Loss of appetite
- Psychiatric problems

Possible Interactions

If you take the following, you should make sure you are taking manganese:

- Antacids containing calcium
- Zinc
- Iron
- Copper
- Magnesium

Anyone taking medications should take manganese only under medical supervision.

Manganese can react strongly with certain drugs. These include:

- Haloperidol and other antipsychotic drugs
- Reserpine (for hypertension)
- H-2 blockers

Liver disease patients should not take manganese, because their condition makes it very hard for the body to excrete the mineral properly.

The Latest News

Another great source for manganese has been discovered in the form of pure maple syrup. One ounce of pure maple syrup will give you 46% of your daily value of this essential mineral. Maple syrup is also rich in thiamine and zinc.

Potassium

What Is It For?

Here is what potassium is believed to be effective for:

High Blood Pressure

The effect on blood pressure is potassium's main function. Potassium supplements can lower blood pressure in people who have a high salt intake.

The best study for this came in 1997, when an analysis was done of 33 different trials related to potassium. Researchers concluded that at least 2,400 mg of potassium daily could significantly lower high blood pressure.

There are also a few more recent studies that reported potassium's effect as being only minimal when it came to hypertension. It should be noted that potassium results could also differ from person to person. Some may show no effects, while others experience a modest reduction in blood pressure.

More recently, the associate professor of medicine at Johns Hopkins University had something to say on this subject in September of the year 2000. Dr. Laurence Appel, MD, MPH issued a report on potassium's link to blood pressure problems. Here's what he had to say: "We have known that potassium is a key player in blood pressure and stroke regulation for some time."[19]

He went on: "...a diet containing approximately 3.5g of elemental potassium daily may contribute to reduced risk of stroke."[20]

Linked with potassium is vitamin B6, as it helps maintain proper potassium balance. Supplementation of 50 mg to 120 mg per day is usually recommended. Likewise, L-taurine in doses of 200 mg to 400 mg daily is useful in combination with potassium. It normalizes potassium flow in and out of the heart muscle.

Supplements that have more than 100 mg of potassium per tablet require a prescription signed by a doctor. This is why most over-the-counter supplements contain just 99 mg. If you are trying to use potassium to help lower blood pressure, it's recommended that you get your doctor's supervision.

What Happens When You Don't Get Enough?

Potassium deficiencies among healthy adults are pretty rare. How do we know this? Well, even in cases where a prescription is given to address a deficiency, the dosage might provide more than a supplement on a drugstore shelf, yet still be less than the potassium one could get by merely eating three pieces of fruit!

Certain conditions can cause a potassium deficiency:

- Chronic vomiting
- Chronic diarrhea
- Taking diuretics that deplete potassium

There are only a few groups that would be classified as at-risk for potassium deficiency. They include:

- Senior citizens
- Those suffering chronic disease
- Those with kidney problems

MINERALS 2

If you're experiencing a potassium deficiency, you may experience the following:

- Muscle weakness, tingling
- Nausea, vomiting, diarrhea
- Fatigue
- Hypertension
- Irregular heart rhythms
- Loss of appetite
- Cardiac arrest, in severe cases

Food Sources

Many fruits, beans, and vegetables are high in potassium. Here's a list of good dietary sources:

- Chard
- Crimini mushrooms
- Celery (raw)
- Avocados
- Squash
- Green beans
- Carrots
- Dried fruit
- Romaine lettuce
- Mustard or collard greens
- Broccoli
- Cantaloupe
- Yams
- Beets
- Fennel
- Bananas
- Cauliflower
- Potatoes (with skin)

- Brussels sprouts
- Papaya
- Legumes (especially lima beans, soybeans, dried peas)

Health Conditions

It's believed that potassium can be useful in treating both high blood pressure and stroke.

Dosage

Typical adults only get about 1,000 mg to 1,500 mg of potassium per day. Now although there is no specific recommended daily allowance for potassium, it's thought that the minimum amount is between 1,600 and 2,000 mg daily.

To control blood pressure, it's thought that a reasonably effective dose is about 3,500 mg daily. The best rule states that you should take in five times more potassium than salt. You have to be careful here though, because the North American diet is naturally salt-heavy. However, a good solution is in getting your potassium from fruit.

Here are regular suggested dosages:

Potassium

Recommended Daily Intake (Men):	1,600-2,000 mg
Recommended Daily Intake (Women):	1,600-2,000 mg
Maximum Recommended Intake:	3,500 mg

Possible Side Effects

Low-dose potassium supplements can cause stomach irritation if you take too many.

Diuretic users should not take potassium supplements.

High amounts of potassium in people who are already healthy can produce adverse effects, including:

- Stomach irritation
- Nausea
- Diarrhea

Excessive amounts can result in more dangerous symptoms and conditions:

- Weakness
- Paralysis
- Listlessness
- Dizziness
- Confusion
- Hypotension
- Heart Block
- Death

Possible Interactions

Those with severe kidney disease or kidney failure should not take potassium or any other supplement without consulting a doctor, as there is always a risk of overdose.

Those taking potassium-sparing diuretics need to be careful about supplements and their fruit intake to make sure they are not taking in too much potassium.

The following medications can deplete your potassium levels:

- Aminoglycosides
- Amphotericin-B
- Fluconazole
- Laxatives
- Levodopa

Anyone taking these medications should take potassium only under medical supervision:

- ACE inhibitors
- Trimethoprim/ sulfamethoxazole

If you take potassium, you may need extra vitamin B12 and magnesium because of its link to other nutrients.

The Latest News

Potassium may play a key role in muscle fatigue. The January 2013 issue of *The Journal of General Physiology* printed a study that looked at the results of muscle activity. In it, a Denmark researcher monitored changes of sodium, potassium, and chloride ions in the working muscles of rats. After activity equaling the legs of a person riding a bicycle for five minutes, an extracellular concentration of potassium occurred that interfered with further muscle stimulation. This result is even more pronounced under conditions of disease or injury.

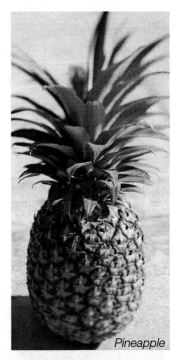
Pineapple

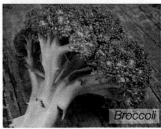
Broccoli

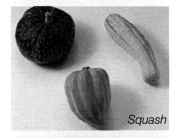
Squash

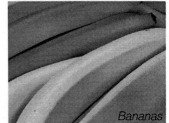
Bananas

MINERALS 2

Selenium

What Is It For?

Here is what selenium is believed to be effective for:

Cancer

Although selenium has been linked to the treatment of many different illnesses, it is linked to preventing only one: cancer.

Even though the evidence is still incomplete, selenium has shown positive results against many types of cancer, especially prostate cancer.

A 1996 study looked at 1,300 men and women who were taking supplements to see how it would affect their skin cancer. While the mineral had no effect on melanoma, it did result in significantly fewer cases of prostate cancer in the men who took selenium versus those who were given a placebo.

At least seven large studies have looked into this selenium-prostate cancer connection. All but one suggested that selenium plays a role in prevention. There are still mysteries surrounding prostate cancer and how the disease starts, so it's also difficult to say how selenium protects against it, we only know it does.

Immune System

Selenium is an immune-booster. Therefore, it's been theorized that it may be of benefit to those with HIV.

Cellular Support

Because of its role as an antioxidant, it's believed that selenium can treat the following:

- Cataracts
- Multiple Sclerosis
- Acne
- Asthma

Other Conditions

Although there is far less evidence to support the theories, it's believed that selenium may be helpful in treating these conditions:

- Arthritis
- Psoriasis
- Ulcers
- Anxiety

What Happens When You Don't Get Enough?

Even though most of us don't get enough selenium, deficiencies in the western world are uncommon.

Of course, sometimes a dietary deficiency will be out of your hands, since so much depends on the selenium content of the soil your food is grown in. Agencies have been created in Canada and the U.S. to monitor this.

Certain conditions can cause a selenium deficiency, such as AIDS and heart disease.

A deficiency raises your risk for the following conditions:

- Rheumatoid arthritis
- Cancer
- Cataracts

When you don't get enough selenium, you are opening yourself up to oxidative damage to any number of your body's tissues.

Food Sources

Some of the healthiest foods are high in selenium. Here's a list of some great dietary sources:

- Shellfish
- Fish (especially salmon, cod, halibut, snapper, tuna)
- Liver
- Mushrooms
- Wheat germ and whole wheat products
- Brazil nuts
- Mustard seeds
- Whole grains (especially oats, barley, and brown rice)
- Turnips
- Garlic
- Orange juice
- Chicken breast
- Pork
- Lamb
- Butter
- Legumes (soybeans, kidney beans)

The selenium content in foods will vary depending on the selenium content of the soil they're grown in.

Health Conditions

It's believed that selenium can be useful in treating:

- Prostate cancer
- HIV
- Cataracts
- Multiple sclerosis
- Acne
- Asthma
- Arthritis
- Psoriasis
- Ulcers
- Anxiety

Dosage

You probably get plenty of selenium in your food. For instance, a three-ounce piece of fish can give you 40–70 micrograms of selenium. Compare that to the recommended daily dose of 55 micrograms. A cup of pasta, rice, or two slices of bread provides up to 35 micrograms. The most selenium-rich food is the Brazil nut. You only need to eat three or four to get your entire recommended daily intake of selenium!

Due to the high dietary amounts available, it may not be necessary for you to supplement with selenium unless you're deficient. If you do supplement,

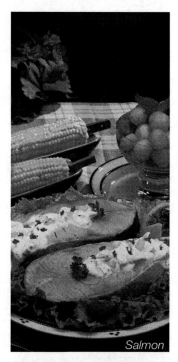

Salmon

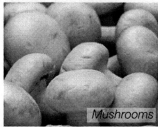

Mushrooms

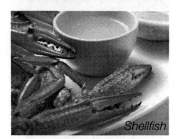

Shellfish

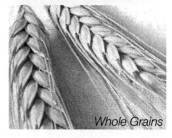

Whole Grains

don't exceed 850 micrograms a day. People who stay in the 100–200-microgram ranges experience no side effects.

Here are regular suggested dosages:

Selenium

Recommended Daily Intake (Men):	100-400 mcg
Recommended Daily Intake (Women):	100-400 mcg
Maximum Recommended Intake:	850 mcg

Possible Side Effects

Selenium can have toxic effects if you exceed the 850-microgram recommendations.

In the worst-case scenario, it can form superoxide compounds that are dangerous.

In less serious cases selenium can produce adverse effects, including:

• Hair loss

• Garlic-like bad breath

• Depression

• Unstable emotions

• Nausea

• Fingernail brittleness and loss

• Upset stomach

• Nervousness

• Weight loss

• Changes to your nervous system

Possible Interactions

A positive interaction from selenium comes in the area of cancer. It appears that selenium can eliminate some of the toxic effects that patients experience when undergoing chemotherapy.

The following medications can deplete your selenium levels or block your body's absorption:

• Corticosteroids

• H-2 blockers

• Proton pump inhibitors

Selenium can negate the effects of statin drugs and supplemental niacin.

The Latest News

The bacteria-fighting qualities of selenium may be a great advancement for implanted devices. Engineers at Brown University coated polycarbonate with nanoparticles of selenium. Polycarbonate is what catheters and endotracheal tubes are made from. Once implanted in the patient, tough colonies of bacteria form what are called biofilms on the surfaces of these plastic devices and become highly resistant to antibiotics. Thus, many patients can develop infections at the site of their implanted device.

One of the best results with the selenium nanoparticle coating was against the bacteria *Staphylococcus aureus*, or staph. Staph infections have become more problematic in hospitals where they are one of the most reported infections. This bacterium has also been increasingly resistant to antibiotics. The good news is that in tests, the selenium coatings reduced colonies of staph by as much as 90%.

Zinc

What Is It For?

The power of zinc can't be minimized. Doctors and researchers alike theorize that zinc can have a beneficial effect in treating many different conditions.

Here is what zinc is believed to be effective for:

Immune System

Zinc supports your immune system in a huge way, due to its virus-fighting capabilities.

One of the viruses it combats is the common cold. It's been proven that zinc lozenges can reduce the symptoms and duration of a cold if taken at the first sign of trouble. For instance, if you suspect your itchy eyes and sneezing are signaling a cold, you may want to use zinc lozenges right away. The zinc will block the rhinovirus (cold) from spreading, while signaling your immune system to jump into action.

Zinc can keep the cold virus from getting a hold in your body and spreading into the respiratory tract. Zinc works especially well in the throat, and it reduces coughing, sore throat, headache, and congestion.

If you already have an upper respiratory tract infection, zinc will still be your best bet. In this case, you can use a nasal spray containing the mineral as well as oral lozenges.

In one trial, 213 patients who were recently infected were given one shot of zinc or placebo nasal spray every four hours. The results were huge. The spray reduced the cold's duration by 75%, and the infection lasted only an average of 2.3 days as opposed to nine days for the placebo group.[21] Other studies have also pointed to zinc's virus-fighting qualities.

If you're deficient in zinc, taking supplements can help you fight off other infections such as pneumonia and diarrhea. It can also reduce the symptoms and improve breathing for those with acute lower respiratory infections.

Because of its excellent virus-fighting properties, zinc can also be used to clear up cold sores, which are caused by the herpes virus. In a double-blind study, 46 people with these herpes lesions on the face were treated with a zinc-based cream or a placebo every two hours. Those getting the topical zinc cream had a significant reduction in both the severity and the duration of the lesions.[22]

Cellular Support

Zinc can help reduce the number of "crises" in red blood cells caused by sickle-cell disease. Because this is such a serious condition, supplementing with high zinc doses should only be done under the watchful eye of a physician.

Skin Health

Most acne sufferers have zinc levels that are lower than normal. While there is no specific proof that zinc can cure acne, studies have shown generally positive results.

Eye Health

Zinc is important in fighting off one of the most common debilitating conditions, that of macular degeneration. It's known that antioxidants can slow the progression of this disease, which leads to blindness in its final phase. Antioxidants such as vitamins C and E and beta-carotene are helpful, but they don't seem to really activate until zinc enters the mix. In fact, zinc is the supplement that, by itself, has been found to preserve vision.

Eating Disorders

Evidence shows that zinc supplements may be useful in treating anorexia. Two smaller studies showed reasonable effectiveness for enhancing weight gain and stabilizing the mood of anorexia nervosa patients.

Other Conditions

Doctors and scientists believe that zinc may be helpful in treating these conditions:

- Arthritis
- Alzheimer's disease
- Attention deficit disorder (ADD)
- Enlarged prostate
- Diabetes
- Eczema
- Impotence
- Tinnitus
- Psoriasis
- Osteoporosis
- Diarrhea
- Peptic ulcers
- Crohn's disease
- Colitis
- Periodontal disease

What Happens When You Don't Get Enough?

Most people don't have to worry about severe zinc deficiencies, but mild to moderate deficiencies can occur. This can happen if you don't take in enough over a long period of time, if your body has trouble absorbing it, if you're losing too much of it, or if you're in a situation where you need an increased amount.

A deficiency causes your body problems in using oxygen, removing carbon dioxide, and generating energy during exercise. If you tire more quickly than normal while exercising, or if you have difficulty gearing up for an intense workout, it could be indicating a zinc deficiency.

Certain groups are more at risk for zinc deficiency:

- Women
- Adolescents
- Infants
- Older adults
- Alcoholics
- Vegetarians
- Those experiencing chronic diarrhea
- Those who have had gastrointestinal surgery
- Those with gastrointestinal disorders

Here are some additional signs that you are suffering from a zinc deficiency:

- More frequent colds or flu
- White spots on fingernails
- Wounds that heal more slowly

- Dulled sense of smell and taste
- Skin problems (acne, psoriasis, eczema flare-ups)
- Low sperm count
- Mild blood glucose intolerance
- Hair loss
- Diarrhea
- Some degree of impotence
- Loss of appetite
- Mental slowness

Since some of these may mimic other conditions, you will want to consult your doctor about supplementing with zinc.

Food Sources

Although it's important that we get some zinc each day, the quantity we need is small, and it's not necessary to eat a huge amount of food to get it.

The most zinc-rich food is oysters. A single serving can provide you with 10 times the daily requirement.

Here's a list of some great dietary sources:

- Oysters
- Fortified cereals
- All meats
- Whole grains (especially whole wheat, oats, rye)
- Nuts, peanut butter
- Yogurt
- Baked beans
- Peas
- Cheese (especially mozzarella and cheddar)

The zinc you get from meat is more easily absorbed than what you get from plant-based sources.

Health Conditions

It's believed that zinc can be useful in treating:

- Impaired immune system
- Viral infections
- Common cold
- Influenza
- Respiratory infections
- Pneumonia
- Diarrhea
- Cold sores
- Complications from sickle-cell disease
- Acne
- Macular degeneration
- Anorexia
- Arthritis
- Alzheimer's disease
- Attention deficit disorder (ADD)
- Enlarged prostate
- Diabetes
- Eczema
- Impotence
- Tinnitus
- Psoriasis

- Osteoporosis
- Diarrhea
- Peptic ulcers
- Crohn's disease
- Colitis
- Periodontal disease

Dosage

The daily recommended amount will give you the support for strong bones and physical energy you need. The upper limits start kicking in at 40 mg, the maximum, since this can increase the risk of a copper deficiency. The dangerous range is about 100 mg and above, if taken for prolonged periods of time. If you need to use zinc long-term, you may want to consult your doctor about adding copper supplements to your routine.

If you are treating a cold with zinc, it's suggested that you use lozenges, and that your dosage of zinc falls between 13–23 mg, every two hours. Use lozenges without sweeteners such as sorbitol or mannitol, and those without citric acid. These substances can reduce the effectiveness of zinc.

If you are trying to treat the following specific conditions, aim for 30 mg of zinc daily:

- Infections
- Colds
- Canker sores
- Sore throat

Zinc is available in different forms, including lozenges, tablets, liquids, and capsules.

If you are going to take zinc as a pill or liquid, look for:

- Zinc piccolinate
- Zinc acetate
- Zinc citrate
- Zinc monomethionine
- Zinc glycerate

These are absorbed well, and are easy on the stomach. Multivitamins are also a good option, since they usually have the proper daily amount of zinc you need.

Here are regular suggested dosages:

Zinc

Recommended Daily Intake (Men):	15 mg
Recommended Daily Intake (Women):	12 mg
Maximum Recommended Intake:	40 mg

Possible Side Effects

Zinc at recommended levels shouldn't cause any problem other than the occasional upset stomach that can usually be solved by eating.

Even if you are upping your dosage to fight a cold or flu, you shouldn't experience adverse effects unless you're taking it long-term. At cold-fighting levels, you might suffer a metallic taste in your mouth, perhaps some nausea and vomiting.

It is only in high doses over long periods of time that the danger of toxicity becomes a possibility. Long-term is considered a period of two weeks or more. At this point, you open yourself up to side effects, including:

- Nausea
- Vomiting
- Diarrhea
- Depressed immune system
- Disrupted copper absorption
- Increased risk of heart disease
- Lowered HDL cholesterol levels
- Risk of Alzheimer's disease

Possible Interactions

There are nutrients that can inhibit your body's absorption of zinc. You should check with a doctor about supplementing with zinc if you take any of the following:

- Calcium
- Manganese
- Soy
- Copper
- Iron

Certain drugs can interact with zinc, and may interfere with your absorption and/or elimination of this mineral:

- Diuretics
- Tetracycline antibiotics
- Quinolones
- ACE inhibitors
- Captopril
- Amiloride
- Oral contraceptives
- Stomach acid–reducing drugs

The Latest News

A new study has linked zinc deficiencies to aging. Scientists from the Linus Pauling Institute discovered a biological mechanism that leads to low zinc in the elderly, followed by a decline of the immune system. Another characteristic is increased inflammation usually associated with cancer, diabetes, autoimmune disease, and heart disease.

As we age, the chemicals that transport zinc to where it's needed are degenerated. An elderly person may be in need of as much as 10 times the regular amount of zinc to fend off the excess inflammation that can lead to degenerative diseases. The researchers recommend a minimum of 11 mg a day for men and 8 mg for women.

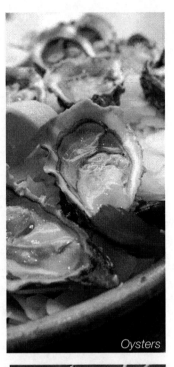

Oysters

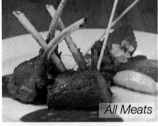

All Meats

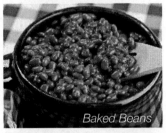

Baked Beans

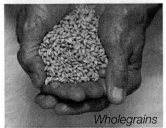

Wholegrains

THE REST OF YOUR ARSENAL: NATURAL SUPPLEMENTS, AMINO ACIDS, AND ENZYMES

Carnitine

What Is It For?

Carnitine is an amino acid that your body manufactures to ensure healthy functioning. It's actually created by a combining of two other amino acids. There are times when your body needs to ramp up its energy production; for instance, when you're pregnant, breast-feeding, or perhaps for athletic performance. At these times, your carnitine levels can get used up, and you may need to supplement them.

Many experts believe that supplementing with carnitine can boost your tissue's energy levels. This has led to the use of carnitine to treat conditions involving the heart and muscle.

Here is what carnitine is believed to be effective for:

Circulation

Carnitine can greatly reduce a symptom of peripheral artery disease called intermittent claudication. It's characterized by pain in the legs, especially when walking or exercising. It's caused by insufficient blood flow when you're resting.

A yearlong study of the condition found that two grams of carnitine daily improved the distance a patient could walk by a whopping 73%.

This is great news for those who have trouble even walking a few blocks due to leg pain.[23]

Heart Health

Chest pain resulting from angina may be reduced by carnitine. Researchers studied 200 angina patients who were given two grams of carnitine in addition to their chest pain medications. Using the amino acid gave them significant relief. Their heart function improved, and they were able to exercise without throbbing chest pain. Another benefit was that their need for the pain meds decreased, along with their cholesterol and triglyceride levels.[24]

The ability to exercise is tied into fighting congestive heart failure. Carnitine can help patients get the exercise they desperately need by relaxing the heart and promoting better pumping of the blood, even in those with problematic ventricles.

Most importantly, carnitine may prevent death from complications of a heart attack. This has been proven. Combining this amino acid with medications lowers the mortality rate among heart attack survivors. The best results occurred when carnitine was given within a day of the attack.

Depression

Approximately three percent of the population suffers from a long-lasting form of depression called dysthymia. While it's not as mentally crippling as more major forms of depression, it can last for years.

A study showed that giving three grams of carnitine to elderly people suffering from dysthymia over a two-month period improved their condition.[25]

Another related amino acid has also shown promise against depression as well as other diseases: acetyl-L-carnitine.

What Happens When You Don't Get Enough?

Carnitine deficiencies are rare, even among vegans. Your body produces carnitine fairly easily.

Deficiencies usually arise due to medical conditions, where your need for carnitine has increased and your body can't keep up. This affects your cells ability to make energy and remove waste and toxins. This can be severe for your heart and skeletal muscles, because they rely heavily on the nutrients transported to them by carnitine.

Certain groups are more at risk for carnitine deficiency:

- Those with rare genetic disorders
- Diabetes patients
- Those with cirrhosis of the liver
- If you become oxygen-deprived (a symptom of some heart conditions)

Here are some signs that you are suffering from a carnitine deficiency:

- Lack of energy
- Irregular heartbeat
- Developing infections easily
- Poor muscle tone
- Gradual weight gain
- Chronic vomiting or fever
- Muscle weakness

Food Sources

Since our body makes it, there is no real dietary requirement for carnitine. It can be found in some foods, mainly in red meat and dairy products. It can be found in the rest of the items on this list, albeit in much smaller amounts.

Here's a list of some dietary sources:

All in the Family: Acetyl-L-Carnitine

Another similar amino acid in the carnitine family, acetyl-L-carnitine does some of the same things as regular carnitine, like breaking down food into energy.

But they differ in that the "acetyl" means that this form helps produce the chemical acetylcholine. This is a neurotransmitter needed for cognitive function.

Because of this extra chemical, it's believed that acetyl-L-carnitine could increase brain function in patients with Alzheimer's disease, depression, age-related memory loss, and stroke. Acetyl-L-carnitine could actually delay the progression of Alzheimer's.

- Red meats
- Dairy products
- Fish
- Ice cream
- Avocados
- Asparagus

Health Conditions

It's believed that carnitine can be useful in treating:

- Lack of energy
- Poor circulation
- Peripheral artery disease
- Angina
- Congestive heart failure
- Complications from heart attack
- Depression

Dosage

There is no dietary requirement for carnitine, and most people will not need supplements.

The dosages listed here are for therapeutic doses. Generally, the dose is divided so that you are taking it three times over your day.

There are no maximum safe levels for children, pregnant women, or patients with renal disease.

Here are regular suggested dosages:

Carnitine

Recommended Daily Intake (Men):	1-3 g
Recommended Daily Intake (Women):	1-3 g
Maximum Recommended Intake:	6 g

Possible Side Effects

Carnitine seems to be very safe in any form.

Occasionally, people have reported the following side effects:

- Stomach discomfort
- Nausea
- Abdominal cramps
- Heartburn
- Body odor
- Seizures
- Diarrhea

Possible Interactions

You may need to supplement with carnitine if you take any of the following:

- Antiseizure medications
- Valproic acid
- Phenytoin

Carnitine can multiply the effects of anticoagulants, including warfarin and acenocoumarol, which could lead to bleeding problems.

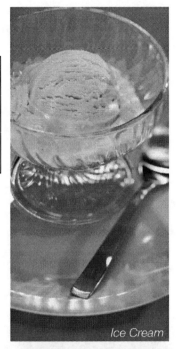
Ice Cream

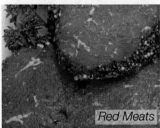
Red Meats

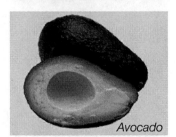
Avocado

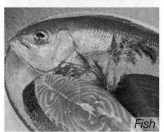
Fish

If you have any disease of the liver or kidneys, it could disrupt your body's manufacturing of carnitine along with other amino acids and enzymes.

Don't mix L-carnitine and D-carnitine; D creates deficiencies of L-carnitine in your body.

The Latest News

Some forms of autism may be linked to a missing gene that controls the creation of carnitine. Researchers from Baylor College of Medicine and Texas Children's Hospital believe that this inborn metabolism error causes a carnitine imbalance. It's unknown whether it is the gene deletion or the modified carnitine that is associated with autism. More studies will be forthcoming. Generally, researchers seem to indicate that a dietary intake of carnitine from birth through the first few years of life will decrease the risk of autism.

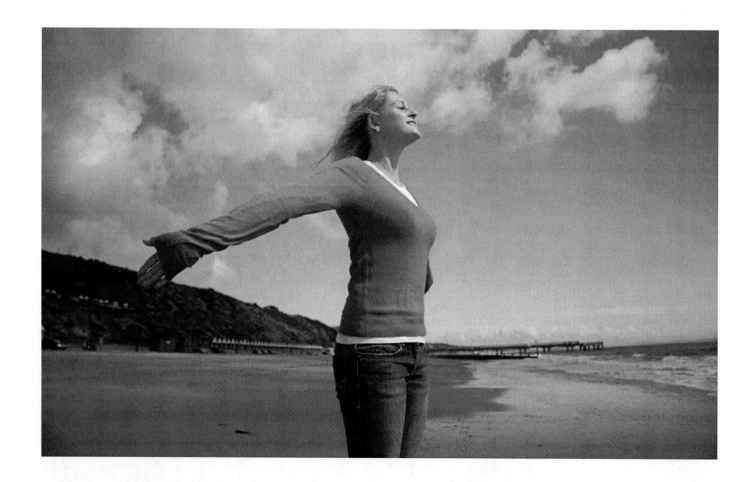

Coenzyme Q10

What Is It For?

Coenzyme Q10, or CoQ10, is a natural antioxidant that your body creates. Its main functions are generating energy, and regulating the oxygen utilization of cells. It comes in two forms, and both are usually included in supplements.

CoQ10 can be found in every cell of your body, but gathers in higher amounts in organs requiring more energy, such as the heart, liver, and kidneys.

Here is what CoQ10 is believed to be effective for:

Heart Health

CoQ10 boosts the heart and is proven to significantly reduce the incidence of heart failure.

Studies have shown that it has led to significant improvements in many cardiac-related diseases and conditions including congestive heart failure, pulmonary edema, cardiac asthma, and has even shortened or eliminated hospitalizations for heart patients.

When the muscles of your heart become diseased over time, it's categorized as cardiomyopathy. This is a very dangerous condition. Small trials have found some hopeful evidence for those with varying types of cardiomyopathy. Patients like these who were given CoQ10 over three years showed improvement. When their treatments were halted, the deterioration started up once more.

High Blood Pressure

CoQ10 can be helpful in treating hypertension. It doesn't cure it, but it does have the ability to lower blood pressure.

In a two-month study, 60 men suffering from high blood pressure were given 120 mg of CoQ10 daily, some received a placebo. While the placebo group showed no significant decrease, the rest had their systolic blood pressure reduced by 10% and their diastolic pressure by nine percent.[26]

Brain Health

CoQ10 levels are lower in those who suffer from Parkinson's disease. Although preliminary, the very first trial examining this link has shown hopeful results. The compound may slow down the rate of functional decline in patients.

In 80 patients, researchers found that CoQ10 can slow the deterioration of the disease, theoretically protecting the area of the brain that Parkinson's damages.[27]

What Happens When You Don't Get Enough?

Deficiencies of CoQ10 have not been widely studied at this time. There may be much we don't know.

The emerging links we have seen to CoQ10 deficiency include most heart problems, along with:

- Angina
- Irregular heart beats
- Hypertension
- Blood glucose issues

- Gum problems
- Stomach ulcers

Food Sources

Just like carnitine, there is no real dietary requirement for CoQ10, since your body creates it. Because carnitine is present in plant and animal cells too, it can be found in many foods.

Here's a list of some dietary sources:

- Sardines
- Mackerel
- Whole grains
- Spinach
- Broccoli
- Beef
- Lamb
- Pork
- Eggs
- Peanuts

Health Conditions

It's believed that CoQ10 can be useful in treating:

- Congestive heart failure
- Pulmonary edema
- Cardiac asthma
- Cardiomyopathy
- High blood pressure
- Hypertension

- Parkinson's disease
- Angina
- Irregular heart beat
- Blood glucose problems
- Gum disease
- Stomach ulcers

Dosage

No severe side effects have been noted for CoQ10, but it's believed that supplemental doses in the 800–1,000-mg range may mark the start of toxicity.

The dosages listed here are for therapeutic doses. Generally, the dose is divided so that you are taking it two or three times over your day.

The compound is absorbed better in an oil-based, soft-gel formulation rather than in tablet form. It should also be taken with food for the same purpose.

Here are regular suggested dosages:

Coenzyme Q10

Recommended Daily Intake (Men):	30-150 mg
Recommended Daily Intake (Women):	30-150 mg
Maximum Recommended Intake:	800-1,000 mg

Possible Side Effects

The side effects of excessive CoQ10 have not been studied. Trials lasting up to six years featuring CoQ10 use found no serious side effects save some intestinal distress. This was true when combining it with drugs, in cases of intolerance, or with what was thought to be toxicity.

Conversely, if you have congestive heart failure and you cease a course of supplementation, your heart condition can worsen. In other words, you might have to take CoQ10 indefinitely.

Possible Interactions

You should NOT take CoQ10 if you are also taking the drug warfarin, without the advice of your doctor.

If you take oral hypoglycemic medications, you may need to reduce your doses of CoQ10 if combining the two.

The following drugs can reduce your body's CoQ10 levels:

- Statin drugs (to lower cholesterol)
- Antipsychotic drugs (from the phenothiazine family)
- Sulfonylureas
- Antihypertensive drugs

- Tricyclic antidepressants

Again, you should consult your doctor when using these drugs about how you can properly maintain your CoQ10 levels.

The Latest News

In a new study, CoQ10 is found to reduce oxidative damage and may slow the progression of Huntington's disease, a neurodegenerative disorder. Huntington's affects behavior, cognition, and movement. It often results in death within 20 years of its onset. It is believed to produce abnormal protein deposits in brain cells that eventually starve the cells of oxygen, effectively destroying them.

CoQ10's ability to reduce oxidative stress could protect the brain from Huntington's, along with its supporting of mitochondria function. Mitochondria are what provide cells with energy. A big study named 2Care is currently underway by the Huntington Study Group. It's evaluating CoQ10's effectiveness in what is the largest study of its kind.

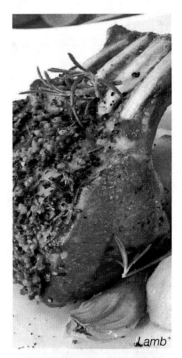
Lamb

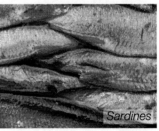
Sardines

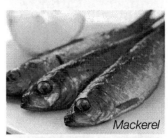
Mackerel

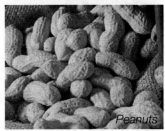
Peanuts

Glucosamine

What Is It For?

Glucosamine is a nutrient your body manufactures to build cartilage, that connective tissue that also cushions your joints.

It isn't found in your food, but you can take it in supplement form. The glucosamine in these is animal-based and is often combined with chondroitin, another substance found in cartilage.

Here is what glucosamine is believed to be effective for:

Joint Problems

Glucosamine combined with chondroitin is now a well-known treatment for relieving the pain of osteoarthritis.

It's known that glucosamine is absorbed well by the body, but the jury on chondroitin sulfate is out. Nevertheless, this is still a popular treatment for arthritis. It won't cure it, but there may be some benefits.

The Lancet undertook a three-year study of more than 100 people with some form of osteoarthritis in the knee. Some were given 1,500 mg of purified glucosamine once daily, the rest received a placebo. Those on glucosamine had an average of 20%–25% less pain than the placebo group. Arthritis was slowed in the glucosamine group, while those on placebo continued to lose cartilage at expected rates. No side effects were reported from the glucosamine dosages.[27]

Glucosamine sulfate relieves arthritic pain as effectively as the most commonly prescribed painkillers. One study found that 20% of knee osteoarthritis patients benefit from doses of 1,500 mg of glucosamine daily. It also helped reduce space between the joints when used over a three-year period compared to those receiving placebo.[28]

In studies like these, even after they've ended, the positive effects of glucosamine can still be seen. While conventional treatments can relieve pain like glucosamine does, they don't have the added benefit of actually being able to slow the disease. Once this is definitively proven once and for all, glucosamine may replace other treatments in the fight against osteoarthritis.

What Happens When You Don't Get Enough?

Deficiencies of glucosamine are tied more to the use of diuretics than anything else. There may be much we don't know.
The symptoms of deficiency include:

- Loss of cartilage
- Joint pain
- Knee pain

Food Sources

Your body makes glucosamine; it's not derived from dietary sources. However, the supplements of glucosamine you can buy are made with bovine cartilage, and the shells of crabs, lobsters, and shrimp.

Health Conditions

It's believed that glucosamine can be useful in treating osteoarthritis.

Dosage

Other than glucosamine-chondroitin mixes, there are three main versions of this supplement, and there are ongoing disputes over which works better:

Glucosamine Sulfate

This form is stabilized with a mineral salt. It is the preferred version, because it is the only one that has been clearly shown to be effective against osteoarthritis.

Glucosamine Hydrochloride

This version has been available longer, and has provided minor benefits to osteoarthritis patients. Its effectiveness has not been studied deeply.

N-acetyl Glucosamine

This version differs in that the combined molecule is larger and more complex than the sulfur-glucosamine or chloride-glucosamine molecule. Your body handles it differently than the other two. More research is needed on this mix, and it's generally thought to be less absorbable than the other versions.

Here are regular suggested dosages, taken three times a day:

Glucosamin

Recommended Daily Intake (Men):	500 mg
Recommended Daily Intake (Women):	500 mg
Maximum Recommended Intake:	Unknown

It may take up to six weeks to begin seeing the effects of glucosamine supplementation, so you need to be patient.

Those who are obese may need supplements to treat osteoarthritis of the knees. In this special case, the formula for supplementing is 20 mg per kilogram of body weight daily.

Possible Side Effects

There is no danger of toxicity with glucosamine. Any problems reported have been minor gastrointestinal distress.

Possible Interactions

There are no known drug interactions with glucosamine.

Patients who take diuretics may need to up their glucosamine levels to make up for any losses through excretion. Higher doses may be needed to regain glucosamine benefits.

There is a theory that supplementing may raise the fasting levels of glucosamine in the blood, leading to higher rates of glycosylation. Glycosylation increases the complications of diabetes. However, there is more proof needed before this becomes a concern.

The Latest News

A huge study called the VITAL (Vitamins and Lifestyle) Cohort wrapped up with some astounding results for glucosamine. This study tracked over 75, 000 participants aged 50–76 who were enrolled between 2000 and 2002. A follow-up was then done with them in 2008.

Glucosamine users reduced their risk of cancer death by 13%. They had an 18% reduced risk of death from all causes. Most astonishingly, they reduced their risk of death due to respiratory illness by a whopping 41%! This was compared to non-users.

Lysine

What Is It For?

Lysine is an essential amino acid. When you see the term "essential," it means that it is a substance your body can't produce; therefore, you need to get it through diet or supplementation.

Your body uses lysine to create protein. It also helps in the formulation of antibodies, hormones, and enzymes.

Here is what lysine is believed to be effective for:

Immune System

Cold sores are skin lesions brought on by the herpes virus. Since herpes is viral, lysine seems to be a good treatment against it. Lysine may reduce the number of herpes flare-ups along with their frequency. Lysine appears to interfere with how herpes spreads and mutates.

Most trials have shown beneficial effects when treating cold sores with lysine. In a study of 52 herpes patients, researchers gave them three grams of lysine daily for six months. Some were given a placebo. Those on lysine supplements averaged 2.4 fewer flare-ups than the placebo group. Flare-ups in the lysine group were also shorter and less severe.[29]

What Happens When You Don't Get Enough?

Lysine deficiencies are unusual, since most people get adequate amounts of it through diet.

However, there are two groups who are regularly at risk for lysine deficiency: vegetarians and vegans whose diets are high in whole grains, and low in legumes, and athletes, due to lysine depletion during vigorous exercise.

If you have one of the rare cases of lysine deficiency, here are the symptoms to look for:

- Kidney stones
- Dizziness
- Loss of appetite
- Bloodshot eyes
- Possible reproductive disorders
- Fatigue
- Nausea
- Irritability
- Anemia

If you have a deficiency, you may also be deficient in carnitine and calcium as well. Losing calcium increases the risk of osteoporosis. If you are unsure, your doctor can test your blood and urine to check your levels.

Food Sources

If your diet includes a regular intake of pastries, cookies, and doughnuts, you are also reducing your intake of lysine. This is because butter and sugar are heated at high temperatures during the baking process, caramelizing the sugars. But what also happens is that any available lysine in the ingredients bonds to the sugar during carmelization, which then makes the lysine harder to absorb.

Here's a list of some other dietary sources:

- All meat
- Soybeans and tofu
- Nuts
- Cheese
- Legumes (beans, peas)
- Fish
- Eggs

Health Conditions

It's believed that lysine can be useful in treating two conditions: impaired immune system and cold sores.

Dosage

You can get this amino acid in many different forms, including tablets, capsules, creams, or liquids, that feature L-lysine.

Most people won't need supplements, but if you do take it, one gram should suffice. Herpes sufferers need a little more, up to three grams, and especially during flare-ups.

Here are regular suggested dosages:

L-lysine

Recommended Daily Intake (Men):	1 g
Recommended Daily Intake (Women):	1 g
Maximum Recommended Intake:	3 g

Possible Side Effects

The side effects of excessive lysine have not been studied. But if you keep to recommended amounts, you should be fine.

Side effects with high amounts of lysine have been seen in animals in the form of gallstones and high cholesterol.

Possible Interactions

There are no known drug interactions with lysine.

Lysine competes with arginine for absorption in the body, so if you're supplementing with arginine, your desired lysine results will be reduced and vice-versa. Arginine may get in the way, especially for herpes sufferers combatting the virus with lysine.

Foods that are high in arginine can also interfere with lysine:

- Peanuts
- Other nuts
- Seeds
- Chocolate

The Latest News

If you are experiencing hair loss, recent studies show that you should be taking lysine. This amino acid is one of the building blocks of protein. Adding plenty of lysine to your diet will help to prevent hair loss, because your hair is also made out of protein. Meat and eggs are good sources for lysine, but you can take supplements too. A therapeutic dose for hair loss would be 500–1,000 mg daily.

Proteolytic Enzymes

What Is It For?

Proteolytic enzymes regulate the function of protein in your body. There are two types: one governs our metabolic functions, the other is digestive and is created by the body to break down dead proteins (cooked or processed food).

When you don't have enough of the digestive enzymes, your body switches over from creating metabolic enzymes to providing more digestive enzymes. Therefore, when you supplement with digestive proteolytic enzymes, you free your system up to support your other metabolic functions.

Here is what proteolytic enzymes are believed to be effective for:

Healing After Surgery

Supplementing with digestive enzymes can help your recovery after a recent surgery. Studies have seen benefits in a variety of situations:

- Bromelain prevented bad bruising in patients who had nasal surgery.

- Bromelain reduced inflammation, edema, and pain in women who needed an episiotomy during childbirth.

- The same results have occurred using different proteolytic enzymes after episiotomies.

- Proteolytic enzymes limited inflammation in those who underwent podiatric surgery.

- Cataract surgery patients had an improved rate of recovery and reduced pain by using proteolytic enzymes. The same was true for knee surgery patients.

Healing After Injury

Enzyme combinations can help to speed the healing of more minor injuries and sports-related injuries.

In a well-designed German study, 44 people with ankle injuries were given a mixture containing all five of the proteolytic enzymes. Their recuperation time was reduced by 50%, and healing was accelerated.[30]

Significant improvements have also been seen with those experiencing a variety of minor sports injuries, including boxers with fractured fingers and facial bruising. The enzymes seem to be particularly good with injuries of this type.

Immune System

If you've ever had chicken pox, the original virus that started it is still within your body. This virus, called varicella, remains dormant in your nerve cells. As we age, our immune systems can become depressed, and this may give the virus a chance to resurface as the painful rash known as shingles or herpes zoster.

Compare to a shingles drug called acyclovir, proteolytic enzymes have had better results in patients with acute cases of this virus, and their pain was reduced. These results were backed up by an additional study.[31]

Arthritis Pain

The most widespread form of arthritis in North America is osteoarthritis. It affects a large part of the population, causing many to live lives of chronic pain.

Proteolytic enzymes have shown to be a great pain reliever for this condition, performing as well as analgesic and prescription drugs. People have reported improvement for chronic neck pain, osteoarthritis of the knee, shoulder arthritis, and spinal pain.

What Happens When You Don't Get Enough?

Deficiencies of proteolytic enzymes are usually tied to changes or conditions within your body, and not to your diet.

Usually the deficiency will be connected to the pancreas, where a disease causes the pancreas to become impaired in its enzyme-creating functions. Your pancreas can be interrupted from forming the enzymes, lipases, and amylases you need to digest food properly. You need to supplement in these cases.

Any of the following conditions can cause a proteolytic enzyme deficiency:

- Pancreatic insufficiency
- Cystic fibrosis
- Chronic indigestion
- Celiac disease
- Crohn's disease
- Stomach surgery
- Pancreas removal

Food Sources

Although all the enzymes are available as supplements, there are dietary sources too. Unfortunately, they are hard to obtain from food for different reasons.

Your pancreas produces two enzymes called trypsin and chymotrypsin that can also be found in food, albeit in minute amounts.

Two other enzymes are found in tropical fruits. Bromelain is found in pineapples, and papain comes from papayas. The catch is, if you want good, therapeutic amounts, you have to eat papayas when they are unripe. Most people don't do this. With pineapple, you'll have to settle for the small amount found in the juice, because the highest levels are in the stem, which is inedible.

Health Conditions

It's believed that proteolytic enzymes can be useful in treating:

- Slow recovery from surgery
- Slow recovery from injury
- Impaired immune system
- Shingles
- Arthritis
- Osteoarthritis

Dosage

There are many different versions and combinations of proteolytic enzyme supplements; therefore, there is no one standard for recommended daily intakes or levels. For these reasons, it's suggested that you follow label instructions closely.

Look for supplements that are enteric coated. The added coating keeps them from being dissolved in your stomach acid, which renders the supplement useless.

Possible Side Effects

Oral enzyme combinations don't typically result in side effects. Some have reported stomach upset and mild allergic symptoms, but these have been uncommon.

Bromelain has been well studied for side effects. Those with high blood pressure need to be very careful with this enzyme, because it can increase the heart rate as well as blood pressure.

Those with certain allergies may be allergic to bromelain as well:

- Wheat flour
- Rye flour
- Kiwis
- Ryegrass
- Grass pollen
- Birch pollen

People with malabsorption diseases should always consult with a doctor about taking proteolytic enzyme supplements. Because they digest and destroy lipases, you may need to take both in order to avoid a deficiency.

Possible Interactions

Papain can potentially exacerbate the effects of antiplatelets and anticoagulants, especially warfarin.

Pancreatin can disrupt your body's absorption of folate.

You should always check with your doctor regarding both of these enzymes.

The Latest News

Some very promising work is being done with proteolytic enzymes and cancer. These enzymes have the ability to break down the walls of cancer cells. However, what usually happens is that these enzymes get diverted from this action by our meat consumption. The enzymes switch over to breaking down meat proteins, which is why we're not getting the full anti-cancer benefits.

When supplementation apart from meals is performed with proteolytic enzymes, they are able to tear the material surrounding the cancer cells, and then our immune system does the rest, treating the damaged cells like any other hostile invader. Amazingly, even terminal cancer patients have benefitted from this action when given heavy doses.

New work by Dr. Nicholas Gonzalez is proving that enzyme supplements may not be destroyed by stomach acids, as was once thought. Dr. Gonzalez is currently using his own specially prepared enzymes along with metabolic therapy on cancer patients in a New York study. He is following FDA clinical guidelines in the hope that one day, proteolytic enzymes will be adopted as a medical cure for cancer.

Quercetin

What Is It For?

Quercetin is one of the flavonoids. Flavonoids are plant-based compounds that have powerful antioxidant qualities.

Here is what quercetin is believed to be effective for:

Immune System

Quercetin is an antioxidant; therefore, it helps protect your body's cells from the oxidizing damage of free radicals. It's believed that quercetin can help prevent cancer because of this quality.

This flavonoid has also shown promise in treating prostatitis. Prostatitis is a condition in men where the prostate gland becomes inflamed. In two of the four forms of prostatitis, this is due to a bacterial infection. The symptoms include:

- Genital discomfort
- Lower back pain
- Abdominal pain
- Painful ejaculation
- Blood in the semen
- Urinary tract infections
- Difficult, frequent, or painful urination
- Fever
- Chills

In addition to relieving pain and symptoms, quercetin may actually reduce the production of inflammatory chemicals. In a month-long study of 30 men with chronic prostatitis, researchers gave them two 500-mg doses of quercetin a day, with others receiving a placebo. The quercetin patients had far greater improvements than the placebo group.[32]

Quercetin has been used to treat hay fever and other allergies. It may stop your immune cells from releasing histamine, the chemical that triggers your defense mechanisms against allergens. It results in irritating symptoms like sneezing, itching, redness, and swelling, sometimes even hives.

Other Conditions

Although evidence is scarce, it's believed that quercetin may aid in the treatment of:

- Atherosclerosis
- High Cholesterol
- Cancer
- Cataracts
- Eczema

What Happens When You Don't Get Enough?

Quercetin increases the effectiveness of vitamin C in the body. A quercetin deficiency may show up in the form of varicose veins.

Food Sources

Here's a list of some dietary sources of quercetin:

- Red wine
- Black tea
- Green tea
- Apples
- Raspberries
- Red grapes
- Citrus fruit
- Cherries
- Onions

- Leafy salad greens
- Broccoli
- Buckwheat

Health Conditions

It's believed that quercetin can be useful in treating:

- Impaired immune system
- Prostatitis
- Allergies
- Hay fever
- Hives
- Asthma
- Cancer
- Atherosclerosis
- High cholesterol
- Cataracts
- Eczema

Dosage

As a bioflavonoid, quercetin is not an essential nutrient; therefore, no dietary requirements have been established.

Supplements are available as pills or tablets. The most easily absorbed form is called chalcone and should be taken on an empty stomach.

Here are the suggested therapeutic dosages:

Quercetin

Recommended Daily Intake (Men): (3 times daily)	200-400 mg
Recommended Daily Intake (Women): (3 times daily)	200-400 mg
Prostatitis Sufferers: (2 times daily)	500 mg
Maximum Recommended Intake: (3 times daily)	600 mg

Possible Side Effects

Quercetin side effects are rare, but include headache and tingling in the extremities.

Pregnant women should avoid this supplement as it's been loosely linked with an increase in the risk of infant leukemia.

Possible Interactions

There are no known pharmaceutical interactions with quercetin. But due to its mode of action in the body, you should be cautious when taking any antiplatelet or anticoagulant drugs. When in doubt, consult your doctor.

The Latest News

Quercetin may soon be used to enhance the performance of athletes. In a study from London's Kingston University, quercetin can increase the amount of the hormone testosterone, which enhances athletic performance. While some athletes have been caught using illegal steroid versions of testosterone, quercetin may turn out to be a legal alternative.

Found in red wine, quercetin is not an illegal substance. However, the researchers are still submitting their various findings to anti-doping boards to make sure this would be an acceptable alternative. Quercetin controls the amount of testosterone excreted in urine, while boosting the body's levels at the same time.

Taurine

What Is It For?

Taurine is a nonessential amino acid. Your body creates it from a combination of vitamin B6 and two other amino acids, methionine and cysteine. Taurine is found abundantly throughout your body, and particularly in your muscles and nervous system.

Here is what taurine is believed to be effective for:

Immune System

It's possible that taurine can treat acute hepatitis cases that are viral in nature. One study gave hepatitis patients large doses of taurine daily in the amount of 12 grams. Others in the group received a placebo. The taurine group experienced a significant improvement in liver function. Although the type of hepatitis in the study wasn't specified, it appears that taurine can keep these cases from becoming chronic.[33]

Heart Health

There is some good evidence to suggest that taurine may be effective against congestive heart failure. One study even said that it was better than coenzyme Q10, which has been more publicly linked to heart health.

The best study looked at 62 congestive heart failure patients. Some were given six grams of taurine daily, while others were given a placebo. The taurine users had significant improvements not seen by the placebo group. Although this study is dated, other smaller trials since have backed up its findings.[34]

Other Conditions

Although evidence is scarce, it's believed that taurine may aid in the treatment of:

- Attention deficit disorder
- Alcoholism
- Diabetes
- Multiple sclerosis
- Hypertension
- Psoriasis
- Epilepsy
- Gallbladder disease
- Cataracts

What Happens When You Don't Get Enough?

Vegetarians and vegans are the most at-risk group for taurine deficiency due to diet. But even they may not need to take supplements as long as they are getting the other building blocks of taurine, namely vitamin B6, methionine, and cysteine.

Some reports indicate that diabetics have lower levels of taurine, but the scientific evidence isn't conclusive as to whether supplements would be beneficial to this group.

Food Sources

There are some foods that contain the building blocks for taurine, but don't actually have any taurine in them. For instance, legumes and nuts contain both methionine and cysteine, but taurine only results after your body's processing plant goes to work on them. This is why vegetarians should always consume lots of legumes and nuts, because they shun the dietary sources that contain taurine.

Here's a list of some dietary sources of taurine:

- Fish
- Meat
- Poultry
- Eggs

Health Conditions

It's believed that taurine can be useful in treating:

- Congestive heart failure
- Hepatitis
- Attention deficit disorder
- Alcoholism
- Diabetes
- Multiple sclerosis
- Hypertension
- Psoriasis
- Epilepsy
- Gallbladder disease
- Cataracts

Dosage

Since the body manufactures taurine, no dietary requirements have been established.

However, if you wanted to treat a medical condition, such as congestive heart failure, therapeutic doses of supplements would be recommended.

Here are the suggested therapeutic dosages, taken three times daily:

Taurine

Recommended Daily Intake (Men):	2 g
Recommended Daily Intake (Women):	2 g
Maximum Recommended Intake:	Undetermined

Possible Side Effects

No side effects have been reported for taurine, and it's considered very safe.

No maximum amount has yet been determined for children, pregnant women, or those with kidney or liver disease.

Possible Interactions

There are no known drug interactions with taurine. If ever in doubt, consult your doctor.

The Latest News

Energy drinks containing taurine and caffeine have been largely considered dangerous for the body, especially myocardial (heart) function. But that opinion may be about to change. Due to the effects of taurine, energy drinks may actually enhance contractions of the left and right ventricles, delivering a positive effect to your heart.

Studies still need to be done, particularly with those suffering from cardiac disease. While caffeine raises blood pressure, taurine promotes a release of calcium from a network of tiny tubes that surround skeletal muscle. When this release happens, the muscle fibers shorten, or contract. In this fashion, taurine helps the heart muscle perform better.

THE BIG LIST:
DEFINITIVE CURES FOR 30 CONDITIONS

Age Spots

The Condition

When certain areas of your skin are exposed to the sun—mainly your hands, arms, and forehead—you can develop what are called age spots. Not to be confused with moles, they are flat and brownish-black in appearance. Years ago, they were more commonly known as "liver spots," perhaps due to their color and shape.

They don't produce any pain, except what you may feel they do to your appearance. They can make you look older and change the hue of your skin. The most common sufferers are those over age 55, but if you spend a lot of time in the sun, they can start showing up as early as age 40.

Although they won't hurt you, age spots are permanent. Some people have opted to remove them via laser treatment or freezing. Sometimes, you can improve your skin's appearance by using creams and lotions.

The Causes

Pigment changes in your skin occur when it's exposed to the sun's radiation or other forms of ultraviolet light. Your body reacts to the exposure by depositing pigment in spots just as it would if you had sustained a bruise or a scar.

Normal bruising can produce the same effect, where sustained pigments of blood get left behind and change the skin color. As we continue to age, we can develop more and more of these age spots.

The Cure

Here are the vitamins that will treat age spots:

Vitamin C:

The antioxidant power of vitamin C can keep age spots at bay, and reduce your skin's signs of aging overall, but not in the way you'd think!

Instead of swallowing supplements, the key is to use this vitamin topically; that is, right on the surface of your skin. There are vitamin C creams available for just this purpose—look for a brand that has 10% of this nutrient.

The antioxidant properties of vitamin C can reduce the amount of sun damage caused by free radicals. Free radicals may be at the heart of much of the tissue damage you can experience, and vitamin C can neutralize them while protecting your healthy tissue from harm.

Vitamin E:

Here's another powerful antioxidant that often works as a team with vitamin C. In fact, if you use them together topically, you can get even better results. Vitamin E can reduce the prominence of age spots, while reducing damage from UV rays. Like vitamin C, vitamin E is available in lotions and creams. Look for one that contains at least five percent vitamin E.

DHEA:

DHEA's full name is a mouthful: dehydro-epiandrosterone. It's a natural steroid hormone that is created by the adrenal glands as they process cholesterol. Research shows that it not only limits age spots, but it also thickens the epidermis (outer layer) and hydrates your skin overall. This one is taken orally.

Avoid age spots the same way you avoid melanoma: limit your sun exposure and make sure to protect your skin. Sun-induced skin cancer is easily the most prevalent form of cancer worldwide, so the value of a good sunscreen can't be emphasized enough. Also, avoid sun exposure during the peak periods of the day, and don't be afraid to wear some protective clothing when you need to.

Vitamins vs. Drugs and Other Treatments: A Cost Comparison

Hydroquinone cream:	$50–$90.00 avg. cost, 30 applications
Laser treatment:	$300+ avg. cost, one treatment
Microdermabrasion:	$75–$300 avg. cost, one treatment
Chemical peel:	$600–$900 avg. cost, one treatment
Cryotherapy:	$600+ avg. cost, one treatment
Vitamin C:	$25.00 or less, 30-day supply
Vitamin E:	$25.00 or less, 30-day supply
DHEA:	$25.00 or less, 30-day supply

Alzheimer's Disease or Dementia

The Condition

There are very few conditions that are as scary as Alzheimer's disease, since the disease attacks the most powerful part of the body—your brain.

It is a degenerative disease that starts slowly, attacking nerve cells as it quietly disrupts memory and personality. As it continues, the afflicted becomes less and less in charge of their emotions, movement, and the ability to recollect even the most recent actions and events. Eventually, the patient can no longer take care of himself or herself.

It's a frustrating and heartbreaking disease with no easy recovery or cure. Alzheimer's-related problems are believed to be the fourth general leading cause of death in North American adults, behind heart disease, cancer, and stroke. It affects many people over the age of 65. As the population of aging adults grows larger, some experts are concerned that Alzheimer's could reach epidemic proportions.

The Causes

Alzheimer's mystifies the medical community, and there is no known cause for this frustrating disease. Some believe free radicals to be the underlying cause, those unstable molecules that cause oxidation to your cells, including those essential brain cells.

Your body creates free radicals as it burns oxygen to make energy. Some of the resulting molecules have unbalanced amounts of electrons, either too many or too few. Once the free radical is created, it goes throughout your body stealing or adding electrons to healthy cells. This causes oxidation that damages the healthy cells, including the many thousands of brain cells you have.

Oxidation has been tied to the risk of dementia, since it is ongoing and cumulative as you age. Free radical damage becomes more prominent because of the natural metabolism of brain cells. It's thought that free radicals may actually kill these cells.

Oxidative damage may also effect one of the central changes seen in people with Alzheimer's, namely amyloid plaques. These hard plaques develop between nerve cells in the brain, blocking the neurotransmissions to and from the rest of the body.

Some theorize that other factors may be coming into play, such as inflammation and even aluminum poisoning. Since no single cause can be identified, it's very hard to pinpoint a single effective treatment.

The Cure

Here are the vitamins that will treat Alzheimer's disease:

Vitamin B1 or Thiamin:

Because of the way it functions in your brain, thiamin may play a role in Alzheimer's. When you have a thiamin deficiency, a result is nerve degeneration just like Alzheimer's. Vitamin B1 also helps the network of nerve receptors in your body known as the cholinergic system. These nerve receptors respond to the release

of acetylcholine, hence the name. A popular Alzheimer's drug also seeks to improve the cholinergic system, just like vitamin B1.

It's important to note that Alzheimer's disease is an incurable condition at this time. No one can truly say whether thiamin can definitely provide positive results in every case, but the evidence would seem to point to benefits.

Studies have been done to see if thiamin can slow down the progression of Alzheimer's. Researchers have seen improvements in the mental function of patients taking in three grams of thiamin daily.[35]

Vitamin E:

There is evidence that vitamin E may also slow the progression of Alzheimer's. A two-year study showed that 340 Alzheimer's patients experienced a slowing of the disease when mega-dosing with vitamin E in amounts of 2,000 IU daily.[36]

Researchers have also discovered a link between the risk of dementia and your intake of vitamin E.

Vitamins vs. Drugs and Other Treatments: A Cost Comparison

Aricept:	$34.99–$199.99 avg. cost
Exelon:	$38.75–$499.95 avg. cost
Razadyne:	$0.91–$11.23 avg. cost, one pill
Namenda:	$252.96–$272.16 avg. cost
Vitamin B1:	$25–$49, 30-day supply
Vitamin E:	$25 or less, 30-day supply

Arteriosclerosis or Atherosclerosis

The Condition

This is another chronic and serious age-related disease, often called "hardening of the arteries." The medical name for it is arteriosclerosis, from the Greek *arterio*, meaning "artery," and *sclerosis*, meaning "hardness." It occurs when the artery walls become thickened, hardened, or experience a loss of elasticity. All these conditions restrict your blood flow.

While the terms "arteriosclerosis" and "atherosclerosis" are often used interchangeably, there are differences between the two. Both conditions affect the body in the same way, but in the case of atherosclerosis, the root of the problem is a buildup of fatty deposits in the artery called atheromas. With arteriosclerosis, calcium deposits, not fat, cause blockage.

When symptoms finally appear for either condition, it is often too late. At this point, the disease has already progressed to the point where it becomes life threatening, with hospitalization and surgery needed to reinstate proper blood flow. People with cardio risk factors can be affected as early as age 30, although the most common cases show up in those much older. This is a slow-progressing disease, and experts suspect it may begin during childhood. Because of this, the sooner action is taken against it, the better.

The Causes

The innermost layer of your artery is called the endothelium. When it weakens, a break can form that allows cholesterols, calcium, fats, and oxidized lipoproteins to enter where they then stick to the artery walls. As time goes on, the buildup can quietly snowball until it becomes a real medical emergency.

Certain activities and conditions make one more susceptible to arterial disease. For instance, in the case of diabetes, it carries with it a great risk of dyslipidemia, or high cholesterol. Evidence shows that type 2 diabetes sufferers may have smaller LDL particles in their blood. These particles are denser, but can slip more easily into cracks in the endothelium layer due to their minuscule size. However, their density makes them more harmful. Therefore, lowering the LDL and triglyceride levels in diabetes patients is recommended to protect them against atherosclerosis.

Another high-risk group are those with hyperlipidemia. Where dyslipidemia includes decreased lipid (fat-soluble molecules) levels in the blood, hyperlipidemia describes increased levels of these fatty substances that can cause hardening of the arteries.

High blood pressure or hypertension is another risk factor. With this condition, the body pushes blood through your veins at harder-than-average rates. The increased pressure can damage the endothelium layer, creating tears or breaks that allow deposits to get inside the artery walls. Strangely enough, atherosclerosis can actually cause hypertension, because your body will attempt to push more blood through the arteries faster to make up for any blockages there.

The Cure

Here are the vitamins that will treat arteriosclerosis/atherosclerosis:

Vitamin C:

High levels of homocysteine create a toxicity that affects the lining of blood vessels. This is linked to the incidence of atherosclerosis. Oxidation of LDL can also damage arterial linings, letting blocking particles in. Vitamin C helps in both of these situations. It's been shown that vitamin C can reverse problems caused by homocysteine.[37]

Vitamin C has also been found to prevent the oxidation of LDL cholesterol and the harmful toxins it releases.[38]

Selenium:

Research has shown that supplementing your diet with selenium can help prevent heart disease resulting from atherosclerosis. One smaller study determined that people who took 100 mcg of selenium daily were less likely to die as a result of heart disease than those in the group that received a placebo. The group consisted of those who had already suffered heart attacks, and the placebo and selenium were randomly given to its members. No deaths occurred in the selenium group, but four people did die of heart disease of those taking the placebo.[39]

Niacin:

For those already diagnosed with heart disease, supplementing with niacin can insure that the condition of your arteries doesn't worsen. Niacin, or vitamin B3, has been proven to reduce atherosclerosis in men at high risk, or who already have existing cardiovascular disease. Those in this group experience fewer deaths, heart attacks and surgeries by taking niacin.

Vitamins vs. Drugs and Other Treatments: A Cost Comparison

There are many different drugs prescribed for atherosclerosis that do different things. Since there are so many, we've picked one from each category to give an idea of average cost:

Mevacor (Lovastatin, cholesterol):	$28.00–$300.00 avg. cost
Plavix (Anti-platelet):	$49.32–$197.42 avg. cost
Lopressor (Beta-blocker):	$100.00–$199.00 avg. cost
Lisinopril (ACE inhibitor):	$32.00–$324.99 avg. cost
Vitamin C:	$25.00 or less, 30-day supply
Selenium:	$25.00 or less, 30-day supply
Niacin:	$25.00 or less, 30-day supply

Arthritis

The Condition

Arthritis is the leading cause of disability in North American adults. It limits the everyday activities of millions of people, and is considered one of the most prevalent forms of disease today. In fact, one in three Americans have some form of this disease, and it seems to be on the rise.

Arthritis is used as an umbrella term for many joint disorders. It comes from the Greek *arthron*, meaning "joint," and *itis*, or "inflammation." The common misconception is that it only strikes the aged, but the truth is that it can appear at any time depending on how your joints are used.

It's characterized by painful, stiff, and swollen joints, usually in the hands and feet. These symptoms are both frustrating and chronic. With time, they can become crippling.

The two most prominent forms of arthritis are osteoarthritis and rheumatoid arthritis. Osteoarthritis can affect the hips, knees, feet, hands, and back, and is accompanied by a deterioration of the cartilage. Rheumatoid arthritis is actually an autoimmune disease that is chronic, and the resulting joint inflammation can spread to other tissues and organs, inflaming them as well.

The Causes

Osteoarthritis affects more than 20 million Americans. It's not an autoimmune disease, but rather starts when there is a degrading of cartilage in at least one joint. Cartilage is the cushiony substance that keeps your bones and tendons from scraping against each other. Osteoarthritis leads to a complete loss of cartilage, accompanied by increasing pain and lack of mobility due to bones rubbing together.

There are some different factors that are thought to be linked to osteoarthritis, like obesity. Heavier people increase the stress on their joints, which speeds up joint damage. However, aging is probably the main cause, simply because with time, you naturally use your joints more and more. This produces a natural wear and tear on cartilage, causing it to degenerate or flake off. Osteoarthritis may also be hereditary, since many cases have been found to strike many members within the same family.

Rheumatoid arthritis is more mysterious. It's hard to track down the cause, since it's an autoimmune disorder that can strike once, never to return, or can be an ongoing series of flare-ups. It causes your body's infection-fighting cells to attack your joint tissues, and can be both chronic and crippling.

The Cure

Here are the vitamins that will treat arthritis:

Glucosamine:

We see this used as an arthritis pain reliever, usually teamed up with chondroitin. It's become very popular and has shown good results. Glucosamine helps in the creation of cartilage.

A large three-year study in *The Lancet* looked at 100 people suffering from mild-to-moderate arthritis of the knee. Some received

1,500 mg of purified glucosamine once a day and some were given a placebo. The glucosamine group averaged 20%–25% less pain than those getting placebo. They also saw a major slowdown in cartilage loss compared to the placebo group, and experienced no side effects from the large dosages.[40]

As a pain reliever, glucosamine has been proven as effective as commonly prescribed painkillers. A study found that 20% of knee osteoarthritis patients would benefit from 1,500 mg of glucosamine a day. It also discovered that glucosamine helped reduce joint space over a three-year period compared to placebo.[41]

The benefits from taking glucosamine are long-lasting, remaining weeks after patients stop taking it. Researchers hope that it won't just relieve symptoms, but play a major role in slowing the disease itself.

SAMe:

In the middle of the last century, a natural substance of the body was discovered named S-adenosylmethionine, or SAMe for short. It preserves the shock-absorbing cartilage that osteoarthritis wears away. It may also repair cartilage that has already been damaged.

The supplement is used not just for relieving joint pain but in the treatment of depression as well. It's usually available in 200 mg pills, and the recommended dosage for fighting arthritis is 400–1,000 mg a day. These supplements are designed to dissolve only when they reach the small intestine for maximum absorption. Like glucosamine, SAMe's pain-killing ability is as good as commonly prescribed drugs.

Vitamin B3:

Although the evidence isn't as strong for this supplement, vitamin B3 (as niacinamide) may be useful in treating osteoarthritis. A three-month study involving 72 arthritic patients showed a 30% decrease in their symptoms after they had taken 3,000 mg doses of niacinamide. Those who had received the placebo actually saw a 10% increase in their symptoms.[42]

Vitamin C:

A dietary deficiency of vitamin C can put you at risk for rheumatoid arthritis. A U.K. study showed a correlation between people aged 45–74 who didn't get enough fruits and vegetables in their diet, and inflammation of the joints. They monitored 23,000 men and women and asked them to maintain a daily food diary. The results were tabulated at the end of each week. This was actually part of a cancer study conducted from 1993 to 2001.

Researchers discovered that 73 people had two or more swollen and painful joints for a period of at least one month. Half of them were diagnosed with rheumatoid arthritis. The lack of fruits and vegetables in their diet had doubled their risk of arthritis.

Those who got the least amount of vitamin C tripled their risk of arthritis, compared with those who had the biggest intake.

The normal U.S. recommended amount is 90 mg a day for men, and 75 mg a day for women. In the study, some were getting less than 40 mg a day. These people increased their arthritis risk by a factor of four. The researchers recommended that based on their findings,

4
DEFINITIVE CURES FOR 30 CONDITIONS

nobody should be getting less than 40 mg of vitamin C a day.[43]

Other:

The search is still on for those substances and nutrients that will prove to be a boon for arthritis sufferers. We know that those with the autoimmune kind are low in nutrients like vitamin E, beta-carotene, and selenium. These are nutrients that have anti-inflammatory properties. Those with low levels of these important substances can increase their rheumatoid arthritis risk by as much as eight times.

Vitamins vs. Drugs and Other Treatments: A Cost Comparison

Prednisone:	$14.00–$167.00 avg. cost
Naproxen:	$18.00–$47.45 avg. cost
Celebrex:	$42.70–$128.49 avg. cost
Glucosamine:	$25.00 or less, 30-day supply
SAMe:	$25.00 or less, 30-day supply
Vitamin B3:	$25.00 or less, 30-day supply
Vitamin C:	$25.00 or less, 30-day supply

Asthma

The Condition

Asthma is a breathing disorder that can be mild or severe. It affects a great many people, whether they are children or adults. Some experts say that the number of asthma cases is rising to epidemic levels. It's the most common chronic illness in children, affecting one out of 15 kids. Asthma strikes about five percent of all North American adults. A combined one million Canadians and 15 million Americans account for an explosion in hospitalization for asthma, which is increasing with each passing year. Sadly, deaths from asthma in North America have doubled in the past two decades from 2,750 to 5,500 per year.

The disorder causes an obstruction of the airways. In an asthma attack, the muscles surrounding your lungs constrict, blocking air from moving freely. The tissues that line the bronchial tubes also swell. The symptoms include coughing, shortness of breath, tightness in the chest, and wheezing.

Many things can bring on an asthma attack, but with asthma becoming so prevalent, some are looking at possible shared factors, such as pollution, climate change, toxins, and food additives. However, there is a lot more research to be done.

The Causes

While we don't know everything about this condition, here is what we do know: all asthmatics have chronic problems relating to inflammation that occurs in their bronchial tubes. Certain triggers can induce an asthma attack in these individuals. The severity of their attack will be determined by how many of these triggers they are susceptible to. Here is a list of triggers:

- Allergens (pollens, foods, dust, mold, etc.)
- Tobacco smoke
- Smog
- Bronchitis
- Respiratory infections
- Aspirin and other drugs
- Pain
- Detergents
- Chemicals
- Exercise
- Gases
- Hormonal factors
- Periods of stress (crying, yelling, panic)

There are other conditions that can increase the risk of asthma. For instance, pregnant women who smoke have a 30% greater risk of their child developing asthma by age six than women who don't smoke during pregnancy. Even children who are not born to mothers who smoke can have a tendency toward asthma where others don't. This may suggest unknown hereditary factors. Your environment and lifestyle also have an impact on your risk for asthma.

The Cure

Here are the vitamins that will treat asthma:

Vitamin B6:

Asthmatics often have vitamin B6 deficiencies; therefore, this nutrient is believed to be a potential asthma treatment. A study was done on 76 asthmatic children over a period of months. The children were administered vitamin B6 doses in the range of 200–300 mg a day. The children were far less reliant on bronchodilators and steroids afterward.[44]

There have also been cases where adults have reported significant improvements taking only 50 mg of vitamin B6 twice a day. If you decide to take vitamin B6 in large amounts, you should first consult your doctor.

Magnesium:

This has turned out to be a mineral miracle for some asthmatics, giving them increased lung function and bronchial tubes that are less reactive to asthma triggers. Injections of magnesium have stopped asthma attacks immediately in patients. Most asthmatics are notoriously deficient in magnesium, so supplements are a good idea. Taking 300 mg daily can prevent spasms in your airways.

Quercetin:

Quercetin is the flavonoid found in many foods, and has been recommended as an asthma treatment. It seems to work the same way as two of the top asthma drugs: "Intal" and "Tilade." It works by releasing the substances that cause inflammation from certain cells in your body. However, while there is scientific evidence for the effectiveness of the asthma drugs, not a lot has been gathered for quercetin. But doesn't mean it doesn't work, just that it isn't as well backed up by studies. Doctors are continuing their experiments with quercetin supplements, which are known to inhibit a specific enzyme that contributes to asthma problems.

Other:

There's still a lot of guesswork and a lot of preliminary evidence when it comes to asthma and natural cures. We do know that asthmatics are deficient in different nutrients. What we don't know is if that can be translated into a specific cure. We can suggest that people with asthma or those at risk for developing it, should fortify their diet with high levels of the following:

- Selenium
- Magnesium
- Vitamins C, B6, and B12
- Fish oil
- Bromelain

Vitamins vs. Drugs and Other Treatments: A Cost Comparison

Advair:	$56.00–$227.56 avg. cost
Symbicort:	$100.00–$300.00 avg. cost
Singulair:	$200.00+ avg. cost
Flovent:	$50.00–$99.00 avg. cost
Vitamin B6:	$25.00 or less, 30-day supply
Magnesium:	$25.00 or less, 30-day supply
Quercetin:	$25.00 or less, 30-day supply

Breast Cancer

The Condition

The most common type of cancer in North American women is melanoma. The second is breast cancer. Breast cancer is an umbrella term that actually describes a number of cancers that affect the breast. Breast cancer develops differently between individuals, with varying prognoses.

Early detection is key when dealing with breast cancer. Women should have regularly scheduled mammograms and breast exams. Between doctor visits, women should do self-exams, with the help of a partner if at all possible. Your partner may be more objective than you are. If caught early, metastasis can be prevented, and the chances for survival can be significantly increased.

The Causes

We don't yet know what causes malignancy for breast cancer or other cancers. When that day arrives, medicine will be forever changed, and perhaps the scourge of cancer can be wiped out. We know how cells become cancerous, but we are still chasing the specific events that trigger a cancerous change. Until then, we need to look to the factors we're aware of that put a woman at risk for breast cancer:

- **History:** If you've had breast cancer, the chances that you will develop it again become greater. If you have family members who have had it, your risk goes up by about 10%.

- **Genetics:** If your cells carry altered genes related to breast cancer, the risk increases.

- **Estrogen:** Your likelihood of breast cancer rises the longer you are exposed to estrogen, either through the body, through a patch, or drugs.

- **Late Childbirth:** Women who wait until after age 30 to have children seem to have an increased risk.

- **The Breast Itself:** A breast with a lot of lobular and ductal tissue is at greater risk for development of cancer than breasts with a lot of fatty tissue. Also, some breasts are denser, which makes it difficult for a mammogram to detect problems.

- **Alcohol:** The more you drink, the greater the risk.

- **Free Radicals:** These are believed to be the culprits behind many cancers.

- **Impaired Immune System:** Poor nutrition, tobacco use, and other factors can depress the immune system, making it harder for your body to kill the abnormal cells that may lead to cancer.

The Cure

Here are the vitamins that will treat breast cancer:

Folic Acid:

Folic acid has properties that can reverse damage to your DNA, so an intake of this vitamin can be important to preventing and treating breast cancer. This is especially true for women who drink alcohol and the accompanying damage it causes.

Studies have shown that when women who drink maintain a diet high in folate or folic acid, their risk of breast cancer is lower than those on low-folate diets. The *Journal of the American Medical Association* conducted a study of women who consumed one-and-a-half drinks a day or more. These women also had a diet rich in folate that were then compared to a similar group that did not take supplements. The folate group reduced their cancer risk by 49%.[45]

Vitamin D:

Breast cancer rates seem to be higher in the areas of the world that aren't highly exposed to the sun. This may be tied to a lack of vitamin D, which your skin creates from UV light. When this vitamin is formed on the skin, it can be "activated" by the liver and kidneys. This form of vitamin D thus goes through a process that is the opposite of cancer cell creation. Active vitamin D may also work against the negative effects of estrogen. Women may be able to reduce their risk of breast cancer by taking more D.

Vitamin D can also be used topically, although you will need a doctor's supervision for this form, due to the potential for toxicity.

An active form of vitamin D called calcitriol is a potent anti-cancer agent that can be added to an ointment. Applying this ointment to the breast can actually reduce the size and potency of an existing tumor!

Coenzyme Q10:

Although no major peer-reviewed journal has tested the link between CoQ10 and breast cancer, there are some studies that have shown it to produce great results.

One study looked at 200 women who were hospitalized for either a biopsy or removal of a breast tumor. A common factor was discovered in the group; all of them had a CoQ10 deficiency. This may not be surprising, since we know CoQ10 is a powerful fighter of free radicals.

A Denmark study reported "remarkable" results against breast cancer. Patients who were given high doses of CoQ10 saw a stabilization of their cancer, and tumors disappeared altogether. The lead researcher said he has "never seen a comparable regression on any conventional anti-tumor therapy." He reported never seeing a two-centimeter tumor spontaneously shrink, and then disappear until administering CoQ10.[46]

Beta-carotene:

A high intake of beta-carotene may reduce the risk of breast cancer for pre-menopausal women. This is especially true for those with a family history of breast cancer, or those who consume a large amount of alcohol.

Vitamins vs. Drugs and Other Treatments: A Cost Comparison

Tamoxifen:	$50.00–$200.00 avg. cost
Arimidex:	$50.00–$200.00 avg. cost
Faslodex:	$50.00–$200.00 avg. cost
Folic acid:	$25.00–$49.00, 30-day supply
Vitamin D:	$9.49–$29.50, 30-day supply
CoQ10:	$13.00–$49.00, 30-day supply

Cataracts

The Condition

Cataracts and the visual impairment they cause are commonly associated with aging. Cataracts are a cloudy area that develops in the lens of your eye. This keeps light from being transmitted properly to the retina. The result is blurred vision, faded colors, or a magnified brightness from glare, lamps, and sunlight. Night vision becomes poor and double vision can result in the affected eye. Cataracts also mean constant changes to prescriptions for glasses. They get progressively worse with time.

The main cause of visual impairment in the U.S. is cataracts. About 1.2 million Americans develop cataracts every year. More than half of adults over 80 have a cataract or have had surgery to remove one. Although you can get cataracts in both eyes, the condition doesn't spread from one to the other.

The Causes

There are a few root causes of cataract formation. The main one is a protein buildup in the lens, which eventually reduces the amount of light reaching the retina. Like a movie screen, the retina then transmits the image it gets to the optic nerve, which carries it to the brain. If the lens is blurry, the retina's picture is blurry, and that's what the brain is given to translate.

In another form of cataracts, the lens simply changes color with age, giving a brownish tint to images.

Experimental studies seem to indicate that there may also be a link between UV rays and cataracts. The UV rays may form toxic free radicals, which then disrupt the lens.

Cataracts that develop early and progress fast seem to be linked to poor nutrition.

Overall, cataracts are considered a natural by-product of aging. If you live to age 60 or more, it's thought that inevitably, you will develop a cataract. However, there are childhood cataracts too. They are referred to as developmental, infantile, or juvenile cataracts. These are due to a molecular defect in the child's genetic makeup. Researchers from the University of Zurich, who found the chromosomal location in the coding region of the gene, first discovered this. Some of these types of cataracts can be present at birth or shortly after. These earliest ones are called congenital cataracts.

The Cure

Here are the vitamins that will treat cataracts:

Vitamin B1, B2, B3:

Supplements containing all three of these can reduce the occurrence of cataracts. Also known as niacin, riboflavin, and thiamin, a person can also derive anti-cataract benefits by upping the amounts in their diet.

Vitamin C:

Even though vitamin C has had mixed results against cataracts, it's probably still a good idea to take it. In a study from Tufts University, a link was found between age, vitamin C, and the risk for common cortical cataracts. Women under age 60 who took 362 mg or more of vitamin C daily had a 57% reduced risk of cataracts than women who took only 140 mg daily. Those taking vitamin C for more than a decade lowered their chances of getting cataracts by 60% compared to those using no supplements at all.[47]

A regular intake of vitamin C is likely to keep you from developing cataracts. In a huge eight-year study of nurses, it was discovered that those taking C supplements for at least 10 years in addition to dietary sources had about half the rate of cataracts as those who didn't.[48]

In another study of 247 women, supplementing with vitamin C reduced their cataract risk by 77%. Cataracts are one condition where dietary vitamin C isn't needed if you are using supplements.

Vitamin E:

Although a little less definitive than the results from vitamin C, supplementing with vitamin E is also linked to reduced risk of cataracts. In several studies, those with low levels of vitamins E and A in their bloodstream were almost twice as likely to develop cataracts. This has been backed up by other reports showing those with the most vitamin E to be the least likely to get cataracts.

Carotenoids:

The source of these is mainly dietary. As children, we were told that carrots were good for the eyes, and today's science seems to back up this old tale.

Carotenoids are the organic colors or pigmentation in vegetables such as carrots, sweet potatoes, spinach, kale, bell peppers and others. These pigments may be effective at preventing cataracts.

In one long study, researchers looked at the likelihood of cataracts in 500 women aged 53–73. Those with higher levels of carotenoids and vitamin C were less likely to develop cataracts.[49]

Two of the carotenoids, lutein, and zeaxanthin, are thought to be specifically linked to preventing cataracts. In one study of U.S. men, they achieved a modestly lower risk of those cataracts that require surgical removal.

Vitamins vs. Drugs and Other Treatments: A Cost Comparison

There are no real cataract drugs available. So, since the only real treatment is surgical removal, here is a comparison based on the procedure versus vitamins:

Surgical Cataract Removal (per eye):	$528.10–$4,461.48 avg. cost
Vitamin B-complex:	$25.00–$49.00 avg. cost, 30-day supply
Vitamin C:	$25.00 or less avg. cost, 30-day supply
Vitamin E:	$25.00 or less avg. cost, 30-day supply

Chronic Fatigue Syndrome

The Condition

Chronic fatigue syndrome is also known as CFS. It's an unexplained persistent fatigue that is accompanied by the following symptoms:

- Sore throat
- Chronic cough
- Allergies
- Sleep disturbances
- Intolerance to alcohol
- Mysterious aches and pains
- Headache
- Depression
- Tender lymph nodes
- Non-refreshing sleep

Technically, fatigue isn't considered CFS unless it's present for six months or more. It's very difficult to treat because its causes aren't known. Medical experts usually try to treat the fatigued body with the use of drugs, supplements, and even herbs to attempt to stimulate the tired patient. In most cases, they are taking their best guess.

About half a million people in the U.S. suffer from some form of CFS. The main sufferers are women, who contract CFS two to four times more often than men.

The Causes

The sad and maddening aspect is that there is no known cause for CFS. Accordingly, there is also no one great treatment for CFS. You can attempt to quell some of its symptoms such as depression, allergies, and sleep deprivation, but relieving those does nothing to eliminate the disease itself.

The Cure

Here are the vitamins that will treat chronic fatigue syndrome:

Magnesium:

Those deficient in this mineral can experience CFS symptoms such as:

- Muscle pain
- Sleep problems
- Depression
- Fever
- Headache

In those with full-blown CFS, increasing the foods they eat that are high in magnesium can reduce muscle aches associated with this disease.

For those with more severe CFS muscle pain, they may need weekly injections of magnesium into the muscle itself. A doctor must administer these.

Carnitine:

Your body uses L-carnitine to convert fat into energy. Any time the energy-producing parts of your cells are disrupted the result can be the fatigue that is associated with CFS. This is why supplementing with carnitine may have benefits to treat CFS.

Many CFS patients have low blood levels of carnitine, and carnitine can even help those whose fatigue isn't a result of CFS.

Vitamins vs. Drugs and Other Treatments: A Cost Comparison

There are no CFS drugs used at this time. Most doctors treat the pain associated with CFS with common pain relievers, like aspirin and ibuprofen, and naproxen:

Naproxen:	$18.00–$47.45 avg. cost
Magnesium:	$25.00 or less avg. cost, 30-day supply
L-carnitine:	$25.00 or less avg. cost, 30-day supply

Chronic Obstructive Pulmonary Disease

The Condition

Chronic obstructive pulmonary disease is otherwise known as COPD. It's a dangerous and unpleasant condition that is a combination of two diseases: chronic bronchitis and emphysema. It affects the alveoli, which are the numerous tiny air sacs in your lungs that exchange oxygen and carbon dioxide. COPD also attacks the bronchial tubes. Both of these add up to obstruction of your airways. Let's look at the two base conditions that make up COPD: namely, emphysema and chronic bronchitis.

Emphysema destroys the air sacs in your lungs and weakens the whole breathing structure. It reduces your ability to take in oxygen and exhale carbon dioxide, and it can cause lung collapse as well.

Chronic bronchitis is characterized by a constant cough accompanied by expelled mucus. Inflammation and lung scarring cause the cough.

You can see how one of these would be unpleasant enough; COPD includes both of them. COPD isn't reversed easily. Smokers are more susceptible: two out of ten smokers eventually contract COPD. COPD mimics other lung conditions as well, but here is a list of additional symptoms:

- Fatigue
- Depression

- Loss of memory
- Confusion
- Restless sleep
- Reduced ability to breathe

The Causes

Cigarette smoking accounts for 90% of all COPD cases. Smoking damages the lungs in multiple ways. For one, it promotes lung inflammation. It also stimulates an enzyme that breaks down the crucial elastic fibers in the lung tissue. Those in the 20% group of smokers that develop COPD should stop smoking immediately. This will prevent the disease from getting worse.

Second-hand smoke could also be a culprit in COPD. It's unsure what the direct effects on the lungs are, but researchers have noticed a link between home environments with smokers and an increase of respiratory infections in the non-smokers living there.

Another cause is thought to be air pollution, although this theory hasn't been concretely proven. The at-risk group would include:

- Construction workers
- Coal miners
- Cotton workers
- Metal workers

One percent of the COPD cases are genetic, caused by a rare deficiency of a certain gene. These cases are hereditary.

The Cure

Here are the vitamins that will treat chronic obstructive pulmonary disease:

N-acetyl Cysteine (NAC):

This is the modified form of the natural amino acid cysteine. NAC works against COPD, but it has yet to be decided exactly how it works. It was originally thought to be effective in breaking up mucus, thereby freeing up the respiratory tract.

NAC reduces the number of acute bronchitis attacks. This was confirmed by a study that examined eight different medical trials on this subject. In this "meta-analysis," an NAC dose of 400–1,200 mg daily reduced incidences of bronchitis attacks in more than 1,400 patients.[50]

Carnitine:

Your body uses L-carnitine to convert fat into energy. With COPD, three different studies have shown that L-carnitine can help these sufferers exercise better. Their tolerance of the demands of physical exertion is higher, and they're likely to experience better efficiency in the lungs and muscles. It means everyday exertions of minimal effort don't cause the shortness of breath that usually occurs with COPD.[51]

Other:

There may be dietary factors involved with COPD as well. If you want to avoid bronchitis and emphysema, your first move is to shun smoking altogether. Your second is to make sure your body is getting enough beneficial vitamins and minerals that can also improve your resistance to COPD:

- Vitamin C
- Vitamin E
- Selenium
- Beta carotene

Vitamins vs. Drugs and Other Treatments: A Cost Comparison

Albuterol:	$25.00–$49.00 avg. cost
Albuterol ipratropium:	$50.00–$99.00 avg. cost
Prednisone:	$14.00–$167.00 avg. cost
N-acetyl cysteine:	$25.00 or less avg. cost, 30-day supply
L-carnitine:	$25.00 or less avg. cost, 30-day supply

Cold Sores

The Condition

These are the sores and open wounds that tend to form around the mouth. The herpes virus causes cold sores, and this form is known as *Herpes simplex*. The *Herpes simplex* group of viruses is highly contagious and cause inflammation. They affect the skin, and can cause various symptoms:

- Burning
- Swelling
- Tingling
- Formation of cold sores
- Open wounds
- Vesicles (fluid-filled sacs)

The virus causes irritating and sometimes painful blisters not just of the mouth, but genital areas as well.

A cold sore might start as a burning or itching sensation near your nose or lips. This is called the prodromal stage. It can progress quickly depending on severity, as quickly as a couple of hours. Blisters can break out and split open, accompanied by a leaking of fluid that crusts over.

The Cause

The herpes virus can quietly reside in your body long before it ever demonstrates any outward symptoms. It can be dormant as it hides in the DNA of certain nerve cells. Once activated, it travels down the nerve to the skin, where it causes a breakout.

Certain events and situations can trigger the herpes virus out of dormancy:

- Stress
- Infections
- Dental work
- Overexposure to sunlight
- Hormonal changes (pregnancy, menstruation)
- Trauma
- Certain foods

The virus may weaken, with each flare-up being less severe than the last.

The Cure

Here are the vitamins that will treat cold sores:

Lysine:

The amino acid lysine can weaken the herpes virus and reduce the number and severity of flare-ups. Since another amino acid, arginine, can counteract lysine's effects, you'll want to avoid the foods containing high amounts of that acid. They include:

- Chocolate
- Gelatin
- Many nuts and seeds

To combat herpes, lysine should be taken in therapeutic doses of 1,250–3,000 mg a day. This has been proven by research studies.

In one such study, patients with recurring cold sores were given three-gram doses of lysine over a six-month period. Others were given placebo. The lysine group had 2.4 fewer flare-ups than those in the placebo group. This is a statistically significant difference. When the lysine group did contract cold sores, they were less severe.[52]

Zinc:

Researchers believe that the antiviral properties of this mineral can help eliminate cases of cold sores. In a double-blind study, 46 sufferers of herpes lesions were treated topically with a zinc-based cream every two hours. Some were treated with a placebo. Users of the zinc cream saw a reduction in the severity and duration of their sores. The topical treatment used was zinc oxide combined with glycine.[53]

Vitamins vs. Drugs and Other Treatments: A Cost Comparison

Abreva (topical cream, 2 gram size):	$16.00–$20.00 avg. cost
Zovirax (topical cream, 5 gram size):	$120.00 avg. cost
Lysine:	$3.00–$12.63 avg. cost, 30-day supply
Zinc:	$5.00–$12.00 avg. cost, 30-day supply

Congestive Heart Failure

The Condition

Congestive heart failure (CHF) is related to heart disease. It's the number one cause of cardiac death in those over 65. About five million people in the U.S. have heart failure, and roughly 250,000 die as a result each year.

CHF is characterized by a decline in heart function, specifically its ability to pump blood into the vascular system. The heart will also experience difficulty taking blood back into itself. This results in a fluid buildup in the lungs and extremities known as pulmonary edema. The heart also enlarges, causing shortness of breath at even the most minor physical exertion. The fluid buildup accounts for the "congestive" part of CHF.

The overall symptoms of CHF are:

- Fatigue
- Intolerance for exercise
- Sleeplessness
- Excessive nighttime urination
- Shortness of breath
- Swelling

Besides vitamin therapy, there are some beneficial things you can start doing immediately, such as eliminating salt from your diet, exercising, and losing weight. You can also make sure that your diet is as nutritional as possible.

The Cause

Medical science has pinpointed the dangerous conditions that will cause congestive heart failure. They include:

- Coronary artery disease (a damaged heart muscle makes healthy heart tissue work harder)
- Previous heart attack (loss of oxygen and nutrients damages heart tissue, which never fully recovers. The heart will always have to work harder because of it.)
- Hypertension (high blood pressure) Abnormal heart valves
- Heart problems from birth
- Hyperthyroidism
- Lung disease

In a nutshell, this means any condition that has injured the heart, where the heart is trying to compensate for an injury, or has had its ability to pump blood impaired.

The Cure

Here are the vitamins that will treat congestive heart failure:

Coenzyme Q10:

This supplement is a strong treatment for CHF, because it can strengthen the heart muscle. It's used widely in a number of countries for various heart conditions.

In a study of 640 patients with CHF, CoQ10 was added to their conventional treatment. Half the group received CoQ10 supplement doses of two mg per every kg of body weight, while the other half of the group received a placebo. The CoQ10 group reported improvement of symptoms, and also experienced significant reductions in cardiac asthma, pulmonary edema and complications that could re-admit them to the hospital. Other studies have backed this one up with similar results.[54]

Magnesium:

CHF sufferers commonly have deficiencies in magnesium, leading experts to theorize that perhaps magnesium supplements can treat this condition. A large study of 14,000 men and women found that higher magnesium content could reduce the risk of coronary heart disease. What is interesting is that this was true for the women, but not for the men.[55]

One important study followed more than 2,300 patients who were given magnesium within a day of experiencing a heart attack. This successfully reduced the death rate.[56]

Researchers followed up with those same patients one to five years later. Those who had supplemented with magnesium had a death rate that was still 21% lower than normal.[57]

Vitamin B1:

Since your heart needs thiamin to function properly, it's thought that large doses could prevent a heart event from tipping over into heart failure. There is no direct evidence to support this theory, but preliminary research has shown that injections of B1 can improve heart function in those who've experienced CHF. Supplements could provide benefits as well.

Carnitine:

In many studies, the natural substance carnitine has improved heart function in CHF patients. Just like CoQ10, it may help treat CHF by reducing damage to the heart muscle. It's also known that CHF sufferers have low blood levels of carnitine.

A major study found that carnitine gave patients a 26% increase in their ability to exercise. In another trial, patients who took one gram of propionyl-L-carnitine twice a day had significant improvements in heart function.[58] A study in 2004 proved that L-carnitine greatly improved the duration of exercise.

Other:

Beneficial study results have identified other helpful supplements in the treatment of CHF:

- Arginine
- Taurine
- Creatine

For conditions like CHF, a healthy lifestyle is key, especially the older you get. Healthy foods can provide much-needed nutrients for your heart. Exercise will also protect and boost your heart. The more sedentary your lifestyle, the greater the risk of heart failure.

Vitamins vs. Drugs and Other Treatments: A Cost Comparison

Accupril:	$50.00–$99.00 avg. cost
Cardizem:	$100.00–$199.00 avg. cost
Norvasc	$200.00+ avg. cost
CoQ10:	$13.00–$49.00 avg. cost, 30-day supply
Magnesium:	$25.00 or less avg. cost, 30-day supply
Vitamin B1:	$25.00–$49.00 avg. cost, 30-day supply
L-carnitine:	$25.00 or less avg. cost, 30-day supply

Depression

The Condition

The psychological disease known as depression is not a condition to be scoffed at, or treated as if a sufferer is merely being "emotional." It is a very real disease and can be very debilitating for some.

The overall symptoms of depression are:

- Frustration
- Anger
- Sadness
- Hopelessness
- Lack of sleep
- Poor concentration
- Hyperactivity
- Inactivity
- Low self-worth
- Suicidal thoughts
- Fatigue
- Poor appetite
- Weight loss
- Weight gain
- Combinations of the above

Depression can cause bodily disruptions, affecting sleep, appetite, and sexual activity. It can cause problems in sufferers more often than people with arthritis, lung disease, and even coronary artery disease.

There are different types of depression. The most common are major depression, dysthymia, and bipolar disorder. Dysthymia lasts longer than other forms of depression, but its symptoms are less severe.

The Cause

Physically, depression is tied to powerful chemicals in the brain that alter or control your moods. Depression is believed to be linked to overly low levels of neurotransmitters or perhaps the brain's inefficient use of them.

Some have a genetic predisposition to depression. In the case of bipolar disorder, it can be a biological vulnerability to depression that gets passed down from family member to family member.

Life events can also be at the root of depression. The death of a loved one can send someone spiraling into depression, or a life-threatening disease that leaves little hope for the future. Such events are powerful enough to disrupt the brain chemistry.

Women are twice as likely to suffer depression as men, although the exact reason for this is unknown.

The Cure

Here are the vitamins that will treat depression:

Phenylalanine:

This naturally occurring amino acid is found in two forms: the "right-hand" form (known as D) and the "left-hand" form (known as L). You can buy a mixed form containing both called D-L-Phenylalanine, and all forms seem to provide relief from the symptoms of depression.

In studies, this amino acid has proven to be as effective as commonly prescribed depression drugs such as imipramine, a tricyclic mood elevator sold under the brand name "Tofranil." It should be noted that the studies didn't compare the amino acid against a placebo.

Acetyl-L-Carnitine:

This is another amino acid that has been researched as a depression treatment. In a study of 60 older adults suffering from dysthymia, they benefitted greatly from doses of acetyl-L-carnitine at three grams a day. Their symptoms were improved over a two-month period compared to those taking a placebo.[59]

5-HTP:

This supplement has been used for decades in Europe as a depression treatment. It can now be found on the shelves of pharmacies and health food stores in America. Although more research is needed, this supplement appears to relieve depression better than a placebo.

In a promising trial, 63 patients with depression were observed over a six-week period. Some took 300 mg a day of 5-HTP while others took the depression drug fluvoxamine. The conclusion was a major one: both were equally effective.[60]

B-Complex Vitamins:

B supplements, especially B12, may help relieve the symptoms of depression, or at least boost the effects of antidepressants.

Other:

Nutritional support is very important when

treating depression. In spite of the fact that it's a psychological disease, diet can actually help prevent it. Healthy eating will ensure that your body gets enough of the depression fighters it needs:

- Vitamin B9
- Omega-3 fatty acid
- Eicosapentaenoic acid (EPA)
- Docosahexaenoic acid (DHA)

Some of these are found in fish oils, so eating fish or taking fish oil supplements can be very beneficial to the brain and nervous system. DHA, for instance, makes up a lot of your brain's gray matter and makes for healthy brain cell function. It forms the protective covering around nerves.

Vitamins vs. Drugs and Other Treatments: A Cost Comparison

Xanax:	$100.00–$199.00 avg. cost
Zoloft:	$200.00+ avg. cost
Prozac:	$200.00+ avg. cost
Phenylalanine:	$6.00–$13.99 avg. cost, 30-day supply
Acetyl-L-carnitine:	$14.00–$57.00 avg. cost, 30-day supply
5-HTP:	$8.00–$43.00 avg. cost, 30-day supply
B-complex:	$9.00–$34.00 avg. cost, 30-day supply

Diabetes

The Condition

When your body cannot control its insulin levels, this is the disease known as diabetes. Insulin is a hormone created by your pancreas. This hormone regulates the amount of glucose, or sugar, in your blood. Glucose provides energy for your body. Insulin stimulates your cells into either storing the glucose when you have enough in your blood, or into converting the glucose into quick energy. When you have insulin problems, your blood sugar can become too high or too low.

There are two types of diabetes:

Type 1:

This form is also known as insulin-dependent diabetes mellitus or juvenile diabetes. Type 1 only accounts for five percent to 10% of all diabetes cases. Just like rheumatoid arthritis, type 1 diabetes is considered an autoimmune disease, because the immune system attacks the beta cells in the pancreas that create insulin. It results in little to no insulin production.

Type 2:

This is more widespread, accounting for 90% of all diabetes cases. With type 2 diabetes, there is no shortage of insulin, but the cells and tissues in the body are insensitive or resistant to insulin.

The overall symptoms of diabetes are:

- Increased thirst
- Frequent urination
- Increased hunger
- Weight loss
- Fatigue
- Blurred vision

Two additional symptoms appear with type 2 diabetes: slow-healing sores or frequent infections and areas of darkened skin.

There are an estimated 18.2 million people in the U.S. with diabetes. That's 6.3% of the total population. Another 13.4 million are considered pre-diabetic; having what's called impaired fasting blood glucose (FBS). Diabetes is twice as common in those over 60 as it is in those who are younger, 18.3% versus 8.7%.

The Cause

Type 1 diabetes results from an unfortunate case of mistaken identity. In this form, your immune system mistakes the insulin-creating cells of your pancreas as invading foreign antigens. Those cells become damaged, essentially hurting your insulin-producing factory.

Heredity is a factor for type 2 diabetes. If someone in your family has had diabetes, your own risk for it is increased. Other factors can also raise your risk for contracting type 2 diabetes:

- Obesity
- Lack of exercise
- A high-fat diet

- High blood pressure
- High triglyceride levels
- Age of 45 or older
- Excessive alcohol consumption

Many of these will work in tandem with each other to bring the onset of diabetes.

The Cure

Here are the vitamins that will treat diabetes:

Chromium:

The anti-diabetic qualities of this mineral are well established, as chromium can improve insulin sensitivity. This is suggested by one study that showed an improvement in glucose intolerance in elderly diabetics who were recovering from an injury. The chromium also helped lower their cholesterol levels, and in turn, lowered their risk for cardiovascular problems.[61]

Chromium plays an essential role in insulin activity but is difficult to obtain through diet due to problems with absorption. So supplementing is a good way to increase chromium levels. Doses of 50–400 mg will enhance insulin effectiveness and decrease fasting blood sugar levels.[62]

Vitamin E:

Diabetes can cause a variety of nerve disorders covered under the umbrella term neuropathy. The antioxidant properties of vitamin E can help prevent these complications. Diabetic patients who take 600–900 mg decrease their fasting blood sugar levels at the same time.[63] Vitamin E also improves glucose tolerance. Those with vitamin E deficiencies are more likely to get diabetes.

Magnesium:

Diabetics are more deficient in this mineral than any other, and supplementation can help them greatly. Magnesium improves the pancreas' insulin production, decreases fasting blood sugar levels, and improves insulin sensitivity.

Alpha-Lipoic Acid:

This powerful antioxidant can operate in both water and fat, where vitamins usually act in one or the other. It was once classified as a vitamin, back in the 1980s. It's a natural compound that has been used for decades in Germany to treat neuropathy resulting from diabetes. It's been found that levels of this acid are lower in diabetics, so supplementing may be helpful. Taking lipoic acid orally or in IV form can lead to great improvements in insulin resistance. Consult your doctor before treating yourself with alpha-lipoic acid.

Niacin:

Vitamin B3 definitely reduces the risk of type 1 diabetes in children, due to its protective effects. For type 2, niacinamide is useful for protecting vital functions and improving glycemic control in adults.

Vitamins vs. Drugs and Other Treatments: A Cost Comparison

Avandia:	$200.00+ avg. cost
Glucophage:	$100.00–$199.00 avg. cost
Actos:	$200.00+ avg. cost
Chromium:	$6.00–$13.99 avg. cost, 30-day supply
Vitamin E:	$25.00 or less avg. cost, 30-day supply
Magnesium:	$25.00 or less avg. cost, 30-day supply
Alpha-lipoic acid:	$7.00–$35.00 avg. cost, 30-day supply
Niacin:	$7.00–$16.00 avg. cost, 30-day supply

Enlarged Prostate

The Condition

This condition can be painful and serious. It's usually seen in men over 50 and is relatively common. It's a growth of the prostate but is non-cancerous. The prostate is a walnut-sized gland that surrounds the urethra, the tube by which urine flows out of the body. When the prostate enlarges, it pushes against the urethra and obstructs urine flow. The wall of the bladder also becomes irritated and may contract more often, even if the bladder isn't full. In an advanced stage, the bladder may become so weakened that it can no longer empty itself.

The medical name for this condition is benign prostatic hyperplasia or BPH for short. Its symptoms are:

- Inability to start/stop urine stream
- Painful urination
- Incontinence
- Urinary retention
- Frequent/urgent need to urinate

The Cause

BPH is a frustrating condition, because we know so little about what causes it. Several theories point to testosterone as a possible factor. Many researchers think that aging of the male reproductive organs triggers BPH. As men age, their production of testosterone decreases, which causes an imbalance in testosterone to estrogen ratios. If it tips too much toward the estrogen side, the prostate gland can become too active, grow, and then become inflamed.

The Cure

Here are the vitamins that will treat enlarged prostate:

Beta-Sitosterol:

This compound has rapidly become a leading treatment for BPH. It's derived from plants like other vitamins; it can reduce inflammation, and may prevent cholesterol from building in the prostate. A literature review examined four previous studies of beta-sitosterol. It showed benefits versus placebo every time, increasing urine flow and the volume of urine.[64]

Now available as a supplement, this compound may help reduce BPH symptoms. The suggested dosage is 60–120 mg. Not only is this a promising natural way to treat enlarged prostate, but beta-sitosterol can also lower your cholesterol levels at the same time.

Zinc:

Zinc is often recommended as a treatment for BPH in both the U.S. and Europe. Taking 30–50 mg a day may reduce the size of the prostate.

Vitamins vs. Drugs and Other Treatments: A Cost Comparison

Flomax:	$200.00+ avg. cost
Avodart:	$200.00+ avg. cost
Proscar:	$200.00+ avg. cost
Beta-sitosterol:	$8.00–$36.00 avg. cost, 30-day supply
Zinc:	$5.00–$12.00 avg. cost, 30-day supply

Erectile Dysfunction

The Condition

Erectile dysfunction, or ED, is a frustrating condition since it affects not only the man who has it, but his partner as well. As ED affects between 15 and 30 million American men, another 15 to 30 million people who are their partners are affected, too. Its symptoms are straightforward: the man cannot attain an erection, or experiences a weak one.

People are desperate for answers to this condition, because it seriously impacts the intimacy of a relationship. Perhaps this desperation is what drug manufacturers seem to prey on and appeal to so heavily.

ED can happen at any age, but is most common in men 65 and older. While occasional problems with poor erections are considered totally normal for a man, a continual pattern may point to ED instead. ED seems to have replaced the term impotence, and men today are more open about seeking help for it. ED is not necessarily an effect of aging, and can actually be treated successfully.

The Cause

ED occurs when any part of the intricate sequence precluding an erection is disrupted. The most common causes of ED are either psychological or the result of medical disorders. Indeed, medical conditions are responsible for more than 70% of ED cases.

Men with diabetes are at risk for ED, since elevated blood sugar can damage small blood vessels and nerves crucial to forming and maintaining an erection.

Likewise, vascular disease can cause reduced blood flow throughout the body, and may be responsible for half the cases of impotence in men over 60.

Other conditions can disrupt the path of nerve impulses from the brain to the penis. They include:

- Stroke
- Neurological diseases
- Drugs
- Spinal injuries

The Cure

Here are the vitamins that will treat erectile dysfunction:

L-Arginine:

The beneficial effects of this amino acid may be linked to nitric oxide, whose creation depends on arginine. An erection requires the dilation of blood vessels; in order for that to happen, those blood vessels need nitric oxide.

Arginine has shown good results in clinical trials. In a double-blind study of 50 ED patients, some were given five grams of arginine

for six weeks, the rest were given a placebo. The arginine users saw improved sexual performance.[65] The high dosage seems to be key, as lower doses of 1.5 mg daily have resulted in no improvement.

Five years earlier, a different study found that six out of 15 men taking arginine experienced sexual improvement, while those on the placebo did not.[66]

DHEA:

The evidence is weaker for the effectiveness of this hormone, but it has been noted that men with ED have had low levels of DHEA. A 50 mg dose daily may improve sexual performance, but the study connected to it has not been well analyzed. However, considering the cost of drugs like "Cialis" and "Viagra," DHEA may be a good option. It should be noted that there is no long-term safety information for this supplement.

Vitamins vs. Drugs and Other Treatments: A Cost Comparison

Viagra:	$200.00+ avg. cost
Cialis:	$200.00+ avg. cost
Levitra:	$200.00+ avg. cost
L-arginine:	$6.00–$39.99 avg. cost, 30-day supply
DHEA:	$25.00 or less avg. cost, 30-day supply

Fibromyalgia

The Condition

Fibromyalgia is a form of arthritis that causes widespread and chronic pain in the muscles and soft joint tissues. Most often, it settles into the neck, shoulders, spine, and hips.

It affects between three to eight million Americans. Because it can easily go undiagnosed, those numbers may actually be as high as 15 million. Although it strikes men and women at any age, eight out of every 10 people with fibromyalgia are women.

The Cause

The causes are unknown, so there are many theories as to what's at the root of this painful disease.

One theory points to metabolic imbalances. In post-menopausal women, some think that a deficiency in the ovarian hormone relaxin might bring on fibromyalgia. Others think a lack of the hormone cortisol may be what triggers the condition.

Poor digestion of proteins is another possibility researchers are looking into.

Since the onset of symptoms has coincided with patients who have also sustained an injury or trauma, some scientists believe the injury itself could be triggering fibromyalgia, perhaps by affecting the central nervous system.

Fibromyalgia may be tied to changes in muscle metabolism, such as decreased blood flow. This would certainly cause fatigue and decreased strength.

Still others believe that a virus or other infectious agent may trigger fibromyalgia, but so far no infection has been identified as the culprit.

The one thing that does seem to be agreed on generally is that fibromyalgia is a disorder of sensory processing, that something is going wrong in the neuroendocrine or neurotransmitter system.

The Cure

Here are the vitamins that will treat fibromyalgia:

Malic Acid/Magnesium:

The evidence for the effectiveness of this acid/mineral combo is inconclusive, but since so little is known about fibromyalgia anyway, this natural treatment may still be worth your time.

In a preliminary trial, 300–600 mg of magnesium was combined with 1,200–2,400 mg of malic acid and the treatment was then observed over two months. It was determined that the mix could reduce muscle pain.[67]

A later study indicated that the mix was no more effective than placebo, but there are bits of research that seem to tie magnesium with fibromyalgia. In 1995, a study was done of the combination called "Super Malic," determining that it was safe to use and could be beneficial to fibromyalgia sufferers.

5-HTP:

Dosages of 5-HTP at around 100 mg three times a day can relieve some of the symptoms of fibromyalgia. This is because 5-HTP raises the serotonin levels in the bloodstream.

There's further good news from a preliminary study. Fifty fibromyalgia patients participated in the double-blind study, receiving 300 mg of 5-HTP for one month. They reported a reduced number of tender spots, reduced pain overall, improved sleep, less joint stiffness in the morning, less anxiety, and less fatigue.[68]

Vitamins vs. Drugs and Other Treatments: A Cost Comparison

Cymbalta:	$200.00+ avg. cost
Effexor:	$100.00–$199.00 avg. cost
Lexapro:	$200.00+ avg. cost
Malic acid/Magnesium:	$9.00–$47.99 avg. cost, 30-day supply
5-HTP:	$8.00–$43.00 avg. cost, 30-day supply

Hemorrhoids

The Condition

This condition is very common, and almost half of all adults will have had a case of hemorrhoids by age 50. Hemorrhoids are also known by the more archaic name piles.

Hemorrhoids are essentially swollen veins in the anus due to too much pressure or straining from bowel movements. Hemorrhoidal symptoms are:

- Burning sensation
- Bleeding
- Pain
- Itching

There are two types of hemorrhoids, internal and external. Internal hemorrhoids don't cause the above-listed symptoms, because the membranes aren't equipped with pain-sensitive nerves. However, straining or irritation when passing stool can damage a hemorrhoid's surface and cause it to bleed.

External hemorrhoids are the painful version of the two. This happens when blood pools in the tissue and forms a clot. Irritation can cause an external hemorrhoid to bleed or itch.

The Cause

Straining while having a bowel movement is the main cause of hemorrhoids. This can occur while having diarrhea or constipation, or if you are just going to the bathroom for a long time. Any increased pressure can cause the veins to swell up.

Heredity can be a factor. If your parents had hemorrhoids, you are more likely to get them as well. Some of the other causes are:

- Obesity
- Heavy lifting
- Pregnancy
- Childbirth
- Standing too long
- Sitting too long

The Cure

Here are the vitamins that will treat hemorrhoids:

Flavonoids:

Some flavonoids have anti-inflammatory effects that can strengthen blood vessels. Citrus bioflavonoids are well accepted as a hemorrhoid treatment in European countries.

The best evidence was found in the study of a product called "Daflon." This product contains the flavonoids diosmin and hesperidin. Other studies have found this treatment effective, even for pregnant women. Patients who suffered continual hemorrhoidal flare-ups used this bioflavonoid combination over two months, 120 subjects in all. They reported a reduction in both the number and severity of flare-ups.[69]

Other studies found it helped relieve symptoms during hemorrhoids, and was beneficial for people with bleeding problems. The dosages given were one to three grams daily.

Other:

To avoid hemorrhoids, a diet high in fiber is highly beneficial. Fiber doesn't have to come from eating just bran either. You can eat fresh fruit, leafy vegetables, and whole-grain breads. Staying hydrated is one of the best things you can do to avoid hemorrhoids; try to drink at least eight glasses a day. Regular exercise is also a big help.

Vitamins vs. Drugs and Other Treatments: A Cost Comparison

Analpram-HC:	$50.00–$99.00 avg. cost
Anusol:	$25.00 or less avg. cost
Nupercainal:	$25.00 or less avg. cost
Daflon:	$12.99–$78.99 avg. cost, 30-day supply

High Blood Pressure

The Condition

As blood pumps through your body, it exerts force against the artery walls, which is called blood pressure. When this pressure is abnormally elevated, it's categorized as high blood pressure.

It's measured in millimeters of mercury (mm Hg). This measurement refers to the height to which your blood pressure can push a column of mercury. A normal blood pressure reading would be 120/80 mm Hg. When your reading exceeds 140/90 mm Hg, you are said to have hypertension. A new category has been added called prehypertension, for readings that fall between the two. Of the numbers, the first one is your systolic blood pressure. This number is the measurement of the pressure in your arteries when your heart beats. The second number is your diastolic pressure. This is the measurement of the pressure in your arteries between heartbeats, or when the heart is resting.

High blood pressure is a warning alarm from your body. If you don't heed this alarm, the consequences can be stroke, kidney disease, and heart disease. This is also why high blood pressure is often referred to as the "silent killer," because you may not show any symptoms at all before one of these catastrophic consequences happens, like a stroke. This is why it is vitally important to treat high blood pressure or hypertension as soon as possible. One in four adults are thought to have hypertension; one in three of them don't know it.

The Cause

The difficulty with this disease is that sometimes it cannot be tied to one particular cause, and often is tied to more than one. There is no complete cure for high blood pressure, but you should still treat it as best you can, with the help of a doctor if necessary. It's not a condition to be ignored.

Some of the causes are:

- Obesity
- Stress
- Family history
- Lack of exercise
- Certain diseases, such as diabetes
- High intake of salt, cholesterol, and fat
- Alcohol abuse

The Cure

Here are the vitamins that will treat high blood pressure:

Coenzyme Q10:

There is good evidence that CoQ10 can help normalize blood pressure levels, as well as aiding vascular function. One study in 1990 showed that CoQ10 lead to major improvements in blood pressure after doses of 100 mg daily for ten weeks.

A follow-up study in 1999 also had positive results. The study ran eight weeks and looked at 60 people supplementing with doses of 120 mg a day. Their average blood pressure was reduced by nine percent.[70]

In a later study, smaller doses of 60 mg worked well to reduce systolic pressure levels.

Potassium:

Researchers have examined at least 33 trials investigating the impact of potassium on blood pressure. The good news is that doses of 2,400 mg daily reduce hypertension.[71] The bad news is that any potassium tablet containing 100 mg or more requires a prescription from a doctor.

Excessive amounts of low-dose potassium tablets can irritate the stomach. If you want to supplement with potassium to combat high blood pressure, you should consult your doctor.

Magnesium:

Prevention is probably the first and best reason to take magnesium. If you are deficient in magnesium, your risk of high blood pressure goes up. There is still a lot of research needed on magnesium, but we do know it has beneficial effects on your cardiac system. Magnesium can also help control your blood pressure, with doses in the 350–500 mg range.

Vitamin C:

At least five double-blind studies have shown that vitamin C reduces blood pressure. While these reductions were only modest, they were still beneficial.

In one of these studies, researchers looked at 40 people who were on drugs for hypertension. They were given 500 mg of vitamin C daily for a month. The vitamin C supplements resulted in a 10% reduction in blood pressure, above and beyond what the drugs were already doing.[72] There are many doctors who recommend one gram of vitamin C a day to combat elevated blood pressure.

Other:

There are immediate things you can do besides supplementing to reduce your risk of hypertension:

- Eat a low-fat diet incorporating fruits and vegetables
- Cut your salt intake
- Exercise
- Lose weight
- Avoid saturated fats
- Maintain good cholesterol levels
- Drink alcohol in moderation (no more than two drinks daily)

Vitamins vs. Drugs and Other Treatments: A Cost Comparison

Avapro:	$200.00+ avg. cost
Norvasc:	$200.00+ avg. cost
Maxzide:	$50.00–$99.00 avg. cost

CoQ10: $13.00–$49.00 avg. cost, 30-day supply

Potassium: $3.00–$14.00 avg. cost, 30-day supply

Magnesium: $25.00 or less avg. cost, 30-day supply

Vitamin C: $25.00 or less avg. cost, 30-day supply

High Cholesterol

The Condition

Cholesterol is a fat created by the liver. It's necessary for our body to function, and all of our cells have cholesterol in their outer layer. Among cholesterol's useful functions is that it insulates the nerve fibers, helps the body metabolize fat-soluble vitamins, and more. When the levels of cholesterol in the bloodstream get excessive, it's said that you have high cholesterol.

When cholesterol is high, it can cause atherosclerosis, or hardening of the arteries. The number one killer in America is heart disease, and the higher your cholesterol levels are, the greater your risk of developing it. Keeping your cholesterol at normal levels also helps you avoid other diseases as well:

- Dyslipidemia
- Hypercholesterolemia
- Hyperlipoproteinemia

Your total cholesterol is made up of the "bad" form, known as LDL cholesterol, the "good" one, known as HDL cholesterol, and triglycerides. LDL causes blockages in the arteries, and HDL prevents buildups. Triglycerides are a form of fat in the blood that can be dangerous.

The Cause

Some of it is dietary. Eating food containing saturated fats will raise your cholesterol and eating unsaturated fats will lower them.

Here's what can put you at risk for high cholesterol:

- Your diet (saturated fats and cholesterol are the enemy)
- Your weight (obesity or being overweight increase cholesterol levels)
- Your lifestyle (smoking, avoiding exercise, being sedentary all raise your risk)
- Family history (your risk is higher if other family members have had it)

The Cure

Here are the vitamins that will treat high cholesterol:

Vitamin B3:

Vitamin B3, or niacin, is the best natural way to bring down high cholesterol. Five different major studies prove that niacin lowers LDL cholesterol by 15%–25%; it lowers triglycerides from 20%–50%; and raises HDL levels 15%–25%. In fact, niacin may be able to control your cholesterol as well as the most expensive prescription drug.

Chromium:

Several studies have shown that, in addition to lowering total cholesterol, chromium may also raise HDL cholesterol as it decreases LDL cholesterol levels.

A double-blind study conducted in 1998 found that taking high amounts of chromium at 500 mcg daily was highly effective in lowering cholesterol when combined with daily exercise.[73]

Vitamin C:

Taking this vitamin isn't intended to reduce your cholesterol levels. But vitamin C's antioxidant qualities will protect your LDL cholesterol from damage by free radicals. This is especially important for those with high LDL levels, as the risks of oxidation damage are higher. The oxidation can lead to hardened arteries and heart disease. Doctors recommend taking one gram of vitamin C daily if you are in this situation.

Other:

There are immediate things you can do besides supplementing to control your cholesterol levels:

- Eat a balanced, nutritious diet
- Get plenty of fiber
- Cut down on cholesterol-rich foods
- Avoid refined foods
- Avoid saturated fats
- Eat whole foods whenever possible

Vitamins vs. Drugs and Other Treatments: A Cost Comparison

Advicor:	$200.00+ avg. cost
Crestor:	$200.00+ avg. cost
Lipitor:	$200.00+ avg. cost
Vitamin B3:	$6.00–$39.18 avg. cost, 30-day supply
Chromium:	$6.00–$13.99 avg. cost, 30-day supply
Vitamin C:	$25.00 or less avg. cost, 30-day supply

Influenza

The Condition

This is an infection of your respiratory system, known better as the flu. It can be caused by any number of viruses, and affects your nose, throat, and lungs.

Influenza is more severe than another infection, the common cold. Influenza is usually marked by:

- Three- to four-day fever
- Lingering headaches
- Severe exhaustion
- Muscle aches

The most dangerous form of this virus is influenza A. It can cause major epidemics, and takes form in many subtypes of the virus, which medical experts monitor annually. They watch the yearly trends and try to predict which form will be most prominent in any given season. Then around each February, they try to create the most effective vaccine.

The severity of influenza A depends on two proteins found on the surface of the virus molecule: hemagglutinin (H) and neuraminidase (N).

The Cause

The flu is highly contagious, and is passed around through what is called droplet spread. When an infected person coughs or sneezes, these micro-droplets can pass through the air, landing on surfaces you touch, or even on your mouth, nose, and tongue. Through contact with these droplets, you become infected.

The Cure

Here are the vitamins that will treat influenza:

Vitamin C:

Boosting your immune system with plenty of vitamin C can prevent the flu. There is research that backs this up.

The 60th meeting of the American Academy of Allergy, Asthma and Immunology presented a study showing that daily users of vitamin C did indeed boost their immune systems. Researchers from Texas wanted to see if vitamin C altered the immune system and if it could provide further protection from viral infections. Subjects took one gram of vitamin C daily, after which doctors examined their immune cells to observe any changes. After only two weeks of supplementing, patients showed a higher level of virus-killing immune cells.

Vitamin C helps your body release interferon. This is an antibody that wraps around your cells, keeping viruses from attaching and spreading. Vitamin C also promotes white blood cell production. These cells are your front-line infection fighters. Last but not least, vitamin C's antioxidant properties guard your immune system from the virus' damaging effects. Adult therapeutic doses range from 500–2,000 mg a day.

Vitamin E:

A 1997 double-blind study looked at vitamin E's ability to boost immunity. A group of 88 people over the age of 65 were given either vitamin E or a placebo. The group was then injected with vaccines against hepatitis B, pneumonia, and tetanus, then monitored for immune system reactions. The results were impressive, with those on vitamin E producing vastly greater amounts of antibodies than the placebo subjects, along with 30% fewer infections.[74]

The Journal of the American Medical Association conducted a 2004 study on vitamin E's ability to prevent respiratory tract infections among nursing home residents. The patients were given supplements of vitamin E over one year to see if immune response truly would occur. Researchers wrote: "We observed a protective effect of vitamin E supplementation on upper respiratory tract infections, particularly the common cold, that merits further investigation." As the flu is also a respiratory tract infection, it's not hard to see how vitamin E could be of benefit.[75]

Vitamins vs. Drugs and Other Treatments: A Cost Comparison

Coricidin HBP:	$25.00 or less avg. cost
Flextra-DS:	$25.00–$49.00 avg. cost
Tamiflu:	$100.00–$199.00 avg. cost
Vitamin E:	$25.00 or less avg. cost, 30-day supply
Vitamin C:	$25.00 or less avg. cost, 30-day supply

Insomnia

The Condition

Whether chronic or only temporary, sleeping problems fall under the condition known as insomnia. Insomnia is nothing to be taken lightly, as it can cause many difficulties besides lack of sleep. Here is a list connected to insomnia:

- Inadequate sleep
- Poor quality sleep
- Inability to sleep
- Waking frequently
- Waking too early
- Non-refreshing sleep
- Confusion
- Headaches
- Irritability
- Immune deficiencies
- Depression
- Fatigue
- General feelings of discomfort, illness, or uneasiness

Occasional insomnia plagues about half of North Americans, and about 20% experience it every night. Insomnia lasting most nights for a month or more is characterized as chronic insomnia. Insomnia lasting from one night to a few weeks is called transient insomnia.

Your likelihood of insomnia increases with age, especially for those over 40.

The Cause

There are many different things that can trigger a bout of insomnia. They include:

- Pain
- Stress
- Anxiety
- Depression
- Use of stimulants
- Prescription drugs
- Heredity
- Change in environment
- Change in work schedule

More severe causes can lead to chronic insomnia. These include:

- Arthritis
- Heart failure
- Asthma
- Parkinson's disease
- Thyroid problems
- Kidney disease

Then there are the factors that will perpetuate insomnia:

- Alcohol
- Caffeine
- Chronic stress
- Worrying about sleep
- Excessive daytime naps
- Smoking

The Cure

Here are the vitamins that will treat insomnia:

Melatonin:

A gland in your brain called the pineal gland produces two hormones that regulate your waking and sleeping hours. During the day, it produces serotonin, which is used to relay nerve signals. At night, it produces melatonin, to make you sleep. When your sleep patterns are disrupted, you may experience a lack of melatonin, and a corresponding lack of sleep. Melatonin supplements can put things right.

Melatonin is often recommended for jet lag. A study compared fast-release melatonin to timed-release melatonin supplements in 300 patients experiencing jet lag. When subjects took melatonin over four days after air travel, they experienced a reduction in fatigue, better quality sleep, longer sleep, less daytime tiredness, and they fell asleep faster.[76]

The hormone seems to be a good solution for all types of insomnia. Here are the situations where it's been tested, and found to be at least marginally effective:

- People working shifts
- Insomnia in elderly people
- Children unable to fall asleep
- Schizophrenics
- People with delayed sleep phase syndrome (preventing people from drifting asleep at a regular hour)

Researchers have looked at situations where the pineal gland delays the release of melatonin due to an unusual sleep disruption. In this case, they were looking at people who stayed up late on Fridays and Saturdays, but who then tried to go to sleep early on Sunday night, with little success. Researchers had them take melatonin supplements about five hours before bedtime and found that their situation had improved.[77]

Valerian Root:

This is an herbal remedy that is often effective when consumed as an ingredient in tea.

Vitamins vs. Drugs and Other Treatments: A Cost Comparison

Ambien:	$200.00+ avg. cost
Lunesta:	$200.00+ avg. cost
Rozerem:	$200.00+ avg. cost
Melatonin:	$4.00–$11.00 avg. cost, 30-day supply
Valerian Root:	$4.00–$13.01 avg. cost, 30-day supply

Macular Degeneration

The Condition

Macular degeneration is the second most common cause of vision loss in those over age 65. Almost two million people in the U.S. will suffer macular degeneration, and with an aging baby-boomer population, those numbers will increase.

With this chronic condition, the most critical part of the retina called the macula becomes injured or deteriorates. This leads to vision loss, sometimes severely. Your central vision may become blurred, or a noticeable blind spot will develop. The peripheral vision is unaffected. Macular degeneration can progress quickly and the damage is usually irreversible. This is why it's important to catch it as soon as possible.

Here are the warning signs of macular degeneration:

- Needing brighter light for reading
- Words appearing blurred
- Dull colors
- Slow increase of haziness in vision
- Blind spot in the center of vision
- Straight lines seem crooked
- Other visual effects out of the ordinary

The Cause

The cause is unknown. We only know the forms in which it occurs.

The "dry" form happens when the macular tissues become thin and pigmentation in your eye is disrupted.

Although less common, the "wet" form happens when there is bleeding around the retina that results in scar tissue. It only accounts for 30% of all cases, but this is the one that can lead to blindness. Theories as to the cause include:

- Diabetes
- Nutritional deficiencies
- Infection
- Head injury
- Genetics

The Cure

Here are the vitamins that will treat macular degeneration:

Zinc:

Important enzymes in your retina depend on the mineral zinc to function effectively. But whether zinc can treat macular degeneration has not been answered definitively. What has been discovered is that zinc can greatly slow down the progression of the disease.

One study looked at people who were already diagnosed with macular degeneration. They were given 45 mg of zinc daily for two years. Their loss of vision was slowed down significantly.[78]

Other:

An unusual study treated macular degeneration patients with a unique mix of vitamins and minerals. The supplement combination included:

- Vitamin C
- Vitamin E
- Riboflavin
- Beta-carotene
- Selenium
- Zinc
- Copper
- Manganese

After six months, 88% of those taking this combo reported improved vision or a halt to the deterioration. Only 59% of the group who didn't take the mix could say the same.[79]

It should also be noted that people with the highest levels of antioxidants have shown the least amount of risk for developing damaging eye conditions.

Vitamins vs. Drugs and Other Treatments: A Cost Comparison

Lucentis:	$200.00+ avg. cost
Eylea:	$200.00+ avg. cost
Macugen:	$200.00+ avg. cost
Zinc:	$5.00–$12.00 avg. cost, 30-day supply

Osteoporosis

The Condition

Bone loss, or osteoporosis, is a serious condition. It strikes about 10 million Americans, with many more unaware that they have it. This is because osteoporosis doesn't show itself until a bone actually breaks. It's considered a "silent" disease due to the absence of noticeable symptoms.

Women are the primary sufferers of osteoporosis. Their bones lose density and begin deteriorating, which can lead to injuries such as hip fractures.

To fend off osteoporosis, you need to strengthen your bones by feeding them an ongoing supply of vitamins and minerals they need. Once osteoporosis sets in, it will worsen if left untreated. The bones gradually weaken until they break. The most common breaks will occur in the hips, spine, and wrists.

The Cause

There are a number of risk factors that can lead to osteoporosis:

- Rapid weight loss
- Smoking
- Calcium deficiency
- Lack of exercise
- Older age
- Small bone structure
- Family history

- Some medications (heparin, phenytoin, ethotoin, prednisone)
- Diseases (endocrine disorders and arthritis)

The Cure

Here are the vitamins that will treat osteoporosis:

Calcium and Vitamin D:

Your bones critically need these two nutrients. They definitively strengthen your bones and prevent osteoporosis. Your body uses calcium to build bone, and vitamin D is needed so the calcium can be absorbed. When these two are combined as a treatment, their abilities to slow and prevent osteoporosis as well as reduce bone loss, speed bone fracture healing, and protect bones from damage due to drugs, becomes amplified.

Remember, though: your body can only absorb up to 500 mg of calcium at a time. Adults over 51 need 1,200 mg daily. Vitamin D should be taken anywhere in the 200–600 IU range. The older you get, the more your body will need supplements.

Elderly people are commonly deficient in both of these nutrients. They will experience a greater number of bone fractures. A study found that they could reduce their risk by supplementing their diets with vitamin D by as much as 20%.[80]

B Vitamins:

The B-vitamins group can reduce the risk of osteoporosis. They appear to lower the levels of the amino acid homocysteine. At high levels, homocysteine can raise your risk for Alzheimer's disease and stroke, and double your risk of osteoporosis and fractured bones.

A study from the Netherlands found this to be true. In a large Boston study, it was determined that men with high homocysteine levels were four times as likely to fracture a hip. Women with high levels were twice as likely. The study involved 825 men and 1,174 women aged 59–91 who were part of the Framingham Heart Study. Homocysteine levels in their blood were monitored for 12–15 years to see how many of the group suffered hip fractures. This injury is the leading cause for elderly people to take up residence in nursing homes.[81]

Taking a multivitamin once a day will keep homocysteine levels at a safe level. Of the B vitamins, the most effective are:

- Folate
- B12
- B6

They can be taken in forms other than capsules, if preferred.

You can reduce your risk of broken bones by eating:

- Dairy products
- Green leafy vegetables
- Carrots
- Avocados
- Almonds
- Cantaloupe

Vitamin K:

Some studies also point to a need for vitamin K. Some of these results showed up in the giant Nurses' Health Study of nearly 13,000 women. Those who had more vitamin K in their diet were far less likely to sustain a hip fracture. Women who ate lettuce daily were 55% less likely to suffer a hip fracture. Researchers identified iceberg lettuce as the best vitamin K source, followed by:

- Broccoli
- Spinach
- Romaine lettuce
- Brussels sprouts[82]

Vitamins vs. Drugs and Other Treatments: A Cost Comparison

Actonel:	$200.00+ avg. cost
Fosamax:	$200.00+ avg. cost
Evista:	$200.00+ avg. cost
Calcium:	$4.00–$13.00 avg. cost, 30-day supply
Vitamin D:	$9.49–$29.50 avg. cost, 30-day supply
Folate:	$6.00–$49.00 avg. cost, 30-day supply
Vitamin B12:	$4.00–$20.00 avg. cost, 30-day supply
Vitamin B6:	$25.00 or less avg. cost, 30-day supply
Vitamin K:	$6.00–$23.00 avg. cost, 30-day supply

Prostate Cancer

The Condition

Every year, 240,000 men are stricken with prostate cancer. With this disease, the goal of prevention cannot be stressed enough, because once you have it, your treatment choices come down to surgery or radiation.

Even though the root cause is unknown, prevention can be achieved. There are a number of things you can do to protect yourself from this cancer. There are certain factors that can contribute to the risk of prostate cancer, and each can be targeted. You can also boost your body's own immunity with cancer-fighting agents.

The Cause

As with all cancers, there are some factors that are uncontrollable. The biggest one is genetics. If your father or grandfather had prostate cancer, your risk for it is dramatically increased.

Another determining factor is race. African-American men are at a higher risk than any other race for this disease. However, Chinese men seem to be on the complete opposite end of this spectrum.

Age is also a major risk factor. Men over 60 have higher incidences of prostate cancer than those under 60, but doctors typically begin watching them at age 50 for any signs.

Some experts believe that carcinogens such as tobacco smoke and air pollutants can contribute to prostate cancer.

Exposure to lead in the environment is another suspect in prostate cancer. There is evidence that high levels of lead and lower levels of zinc and copper have been found in men with prostate cancer. Lead may act as a block against the absorption of zinc and copper, and aggravate prostate cancer.

The Cure

Here are the vitamins that will treat prostate cancer:

Selenium and Vitamin E:

Boosting your levels of selenium has been clinically proven to help protect against prostate cancer. *The British Journal of Cancer* examined 13 years worth of trial research on selenium and cancer, particularly in those patients with selenium deficiencies. Their conclusion was that selenium enables normal cell death in the prostate, and blocks the development of new blood cells, thereby halting the spread of cancerous cells in the prostate altogether.[83]

Another study links selenium levels in the body and prostate cancer. Researchers found that men with higher levels of selenium were far less likely to contract the disease than other men. It was suggested that selenium is a useful tool in lowering the risk of contracting this cancer.[84]

A huge study called "SELECT" is currently underway that will definitively identify selenium as a prostate cancer treatment. It's also looking at the combination of selenium and vitamin E.

As a treatment for prostate cancer, it's suggested that you consult your doctor.

Lycopene:

This natural antioxidant has been linked to a reduced risk for prostate cancer. It's found in many fruits and vegetables, especially tomatoes. Men who eat at least six mg of lycopene daily reduce their cancer risk significantly. While lycopene as a supplement has not been widely studied, the benefits men get from dietary lycopene cannot be ignored. Men should get as much as they can, whether their tomatoes are raw or cooked.

Vitamins vs. Drugs and Other Treatments: A Cost Comparison

Casodex:	$200.00+ avg. cost
Cytoxan:	$200.00+ avg. cost
Firmagon:	$200.00+ avg. cost
Selenium:	$4.00–$18.00 avg. cost, 30-day supply
Vitamin E:	$25.00 or less avg. cost, 30-day supply
Lycopene:	$8.00–$54.00 avg. cost, 30-day supply

Shingles

The Condition

The virus that gives you chicken pox as a kid may show up later in life to give you shingles as an adult. In fact, almost 90% of those who've had chicken pox are at risk of developing shingles because of the *Herpes zoster* virus.

A member of this herpes virus family is called the varicella virus. It can lie dormant in the body until it is triggered by a weakened immune system, resulting in a case of shingles. The symptoms of shingles are:

- Tingling
- Shooting pain
- Itchiness around an area of skin
- Rash, or rash accompanied by severe pain
- Blisters

The Cause

The varicella virus is of the same viral family responsible for cold sores and genital herpes. These viruses lie in wait in the nervous system after the initial infection. This happens if your immune system doesn't completely destroy the virus after chicken pox occurs. What remains in your body can re-emerge in later years, speeding along the nerve pathways to the skin, causing a shingles outbreak. Elderly people and those with weakened immune systems are the most at-risk groups.

The Cure

Here are the vitamins that will treat shingles:

Proteolytic Enzymes:

Vitamins E and B12 have both been suggested for treating shingles, but the evidence so far hasn't been overwhelming. However, proteolytic enzymes are the best natural way to relieve shingles. Not only are these enzymes beneficial for their protective effects on the pancreas, but they may also treat acute cases of the *Herpes zoster* virus when taken orally.

In a two-week double-blind study of 190 shingles patients, proteolytic enzymes were administered at 20 capsules a day. These capsules contained 30 mg of trypsin, 30 mg of chymotrypsin, and 75 mg of papain. Compared to the leading antiviral drug acyclovir, the proteolytic enzymes provided the same amount of pain relief, but fewer side effects than the drug. The drug also had the side effect of stomach disturbances.[85] Other studies have had similar findings.

Vitamins vs. Drugs and Other Treatments: A Cost Comparison

Acyclovir:	$100.00–$199.00 avg. cost
Valtrex:	$200.00+ avg. cost
Famvir:	$100.00–$199.00 avg. cost
Proteolytic enzymes:	$17.00–$97.20 avg. cost, 30-day supply

Sinusitis

The Condition

Sinuses are air pockets within the bones of your face and skull. They connect to your nasal passages via small tubes and channels. The channels allow air to pass through the nose and into the sinuses. They also allow the mucus from the sinus cavities to flow into the nose, where you expel it. When the sinuses become infected or inflamed, it results in the condition known as sinusitis.

Acute cases of sinusitis last up to three weeks, and chronic cases can last up to two months or longer. Sinusitis can also be recurrent, popping up multiple times in the course of a year. About 37 million Americans contract sinusitis every year. Here are symptoms associated with sinusitis:

- Morning headaches
- Jaw pain
- Tooth pain
- Eye swelling
- Eye pain
- Earaches
- Neck pain
- Fatigue
- Fever
- Cough
- Sore throat

- Loss of smell
- Runny nose
- Severe nasal congestion

Your immune system is your first line of defense. If it is strong, you are better able to fight off infections and colds.

The Cause

In acute cases of sinusitis, the culprit is usually an infection of the upper respiratory tract. This infection may be in the form of a virus, bacteria, or fungus, such as those that cause the common cold and flu. The mucous membranes in the nose then swell up, which blocks the sinus openings. Once blocked off, bacteria trapped within the sinuses grow.

Allergies can cause this type of blockage as can other conditions such as a deviated nasal septum (crooked nostrils) or nasal polyps (growths of tissue in the nasal passage).

Cases are designated as chronic when the small openings that drain mucus from the sinuses are blocked. Chronic means they are recurring. The causes are the same as those for acute cases, but the chronic cases return more easily and often.

The Cure

Here are the vitamins that will treat sinusitis:

Bromelain:

This is the enzyme found in pineapples. It's reported to relieve sinusitis by reducing mucus buildup in the sinuses. In one double-blind study, bromelain provided good to excellent results for 87% of those taking it to cure their sinusitis.[86] Other studies have revealed similar benefits.

When taking bromelain tablets, look for enteric-coated tablets. The coating prevents your stomach acids from destroying the bromelain before your body can absorb it.

Vitamins vs. Drugs and Other Treatments: A Cost Comparison

Cefzil:	$100.00–$199.00 avg. cost
Cipro:	$100.00–$199.00 avg. cost
Zithromax:	$100.00–$199.00 avg. cost
Bromelain:	$8.00–$23.00 avg. cost, 30-day supply

Sore Throat

The Condition

If you've had a cold, you're probably all too familiar with that miserable achy feeling you get at the back of your throat. It may be a dull ache, or an irritation that causes you to cough constantly until every cough hurts. The pain is usually concentrated around the tonsils and can cause difficulty swallowing, along with swelling in the throat and glands.

If your immune system is boosted by a healthy intake of nutrients, it can help you avoid getting a sore throat as well as colds and flu.

The Cause

There are multiple causes for sore throat, and it is often referred to as a symptom for other conditions, such as colds and flu.

In some cases, it is a result of tonsillitis. This is when the tonsils become inflamed, and it causes a deep soreness in the throat. Sometimes the tonsils need to be removed altogether.

A sore throat can result from a bacterial infection. One of the more well-known bacterial infections is called strep, short for the bacteria streptococcus. Antibiotics can clear up strep throat, but taking too many antibiotics is damaging to your system, so you may want to have your doctor do a culture, or swab, of your throat to recommend the best treatment.

Your voice box can become infected, too, causing swelling. Infections in this area are more dangerous and require immediate medical attention.

Sore throat can be viral in nature too, and in these cases, you may just need to wait until the virus subsides. There are some things you can take to alleviate your symptoms.

The Cure

Here are the vitamins that will treat a sore throat:

Zinc:

The benefits of zinc have become so widely recognized that you now see it as a regular component in many cough drop formulations. Zinc is also recognized as a great cold fighter.

A study found that zinc might interfere with the reproduction of viral cells, in addition to relieving cold symptoms and bolstering the immune system.[87]

Another double-blind randomized study was done with both adults and children participating. It was found that zinc lozenges reduced the duration of colds and reduced the severity of their symptoms, including sore throat and cough.[88]

A third trial was also randomized and controlled, but it was even more in-depth. It found that compared to placebo, zinc lozenges could reduce a cold's duration by seven days. The researchers created two groups, giving one a double dose of 23 mg in a zinc lozenge to suck on after waking, and then an additional 23-mg zinc lozenge every two hours. The other group followed the same instructions, but the lozenge was a placebo. After a week, 87% of the zinc users had no more symptoms. Only 46% of the placebo group reported similar results.

Vitamins vs. Drugs and Other Treatments: A Cost Comparison

Cefzil:	$100.00–$199.00 avg. cost
Amoxil:	$25.00 or less avg. cost
Ceftin:	$100.00–$199.00 avg. cost
Zinc:	$5.00–$12.00 avg. cost, 30-day supply

Tinnitus

The Condition

Also known as "ringing of the ears," tinnitus is a common condition. It describes a persistent sound in the ears that can take different forms:

- Buzzing
- Roaring
- Whistling
- Ringing
- Hissing
- Pulsing
- Loudness

Tinnitus can be continuous or intermittent. It can result from a loud noise nearby, like a gunshot or explosion, and the ringing can subside after a few days. But for others, it is a chronic condition that can become serious. Tinnitus is not only annoying; it can also cause insomnia and disrupt sleep patterns.

The Cause

Excessive noise can damage the ear, resulting in tinnitus. This can happen after attending concerts, or even by standing too close to a speaker or instrument. Tinnitus may also result from an irritated nerve.

There are rare cases where a vein inside the ear becomes enlarged, and your tinnitus is actually the sound of blood rushing through it. In this case, it may require serious treatment.

If your tinnitus persists for days, especially after a damaging noise event, you may need to be diagnosed by a doctor.

The Cure

Here are the vitamins that will treat tinnitus:

Vitamin A:

Also known as retinoic acid, vitamin A is known to be very effective in healing cells in the inner ear called epithelial cells. Some evidence is also promising for topical applications of vitamin A that may help heal damage to the ear.

An award-winning study has shown that hair cells within the inner ear can be regenerated and repaired by a combination of vitamin A and growth hormones.[90]

In another study, cod liver oil was applied to damaged ears. The result was significantly faster healing than patients treated with a placebo or saline. The conclusion was that the vitamin A in the cod liver oil could be the active ingredient that heals ear damage.[91]

Zinc:

Correcting a zinc deficiency can also reduce the symptoms of tinnitus and treat hearing loss. This is done primarily for elderly patients, but there's no reason to believe other age groups couldn't also benefit.

A trial of people with low zinc levels showed great results after they were given high doses (50 mg) of zinc daily, a zinc-related substance, or a placebo for two months. Nearly 50% of the zinc patients had clinically significant improvements in their tinnitus symptoms. There was a subjective lessening of symptoms in 82% of subjects. In the zinc-related group, the average severity of symptoms was reduced by 46%. The placebo group showed no significant improvements.[92]

Since high doses of zinc can be dangerous, it is important to consult your doctor before starting any supplementation.

Melatonin:

This hormone can also improve symptoms of tinnitus. One double-blind trial administered three milligrams of melatonin nightly for over a month. It improved tinnitus symptoms slightly for all, but was more effective for those who had tinnitus in both ears. After one month, improvements were reported in 47% of those who experienced disturbed sleep due to tinnitus. Of the placebo group, only 20% reported improvements.[93]

Vitamins vs. Drugs and Other Treatments: A Cost Comparison

Xanax:	$100.00–$199.00 avg. cost
Pamelor:	$25.00 or less avg. cost
Niravam:	$100.00–$199.00 avg. cost
Vitamin A:	$3.00–$14.00 avg. cost, 30-day supply
Zinc:	$5.00–$12.00 avg. cost, 30-day supply
Melatonin:	$4.00–$11.00 avg. cost, 30-day supply

Urinary Tract Infection

The Condition

This is a bacterial infection affecting the tube (the urethra) that carries urine out of your body. It can also affect your bladder, which holds the urine. It is a common infection that can be painful and even dangerous to your kidneys if left untreated. Here are some of the symptoms associated with a urinary tract infection:

- Frequent or urgent need to urinate
- Burning sensation during urination
- Sensation of inability to urinate
- Blood in the urine
- Abdominal cramps

The Cause

There can be many reasons for developing a urinary tract infection, the most common being a depressed immune system. This can happen due to a lack of nutrients, or these other causes:

- Overuse of antibiotics
- Auto-immune disease
- Diabetes
- Pregnancy

A weakened immune system can allow bacteria to breed unchecked. Some of the bacteria that can cause urinary tract infection are *Escherichia coli* (E. coli), *Pseudomonas aeruginosa*, or *Staphylococcus saprophyticus* (staph).

The Cure

Here are the vitamins that will treat a urinary tract infection:

Vitamin C:

If the infection is caught early enough, vitamin C is highly effective in killing infectious bacteria. It's 100% natural, and bacteria can't stand up to its super-acidic properties.

One study looked at various bacteria fighters and their link to treating infection. One of these is nitrite, which is produced in urine at early stages of infection to kill invading bacteria. Researchers found that when they combined it with vitamin C, the nitrite was stronger and more potent. The growth of three major bacteria that cause urinary tract infection were significantly reduced by the nitrite, and then reduced even further with the addition of vitamin C. The vitamin appears to raise acidity in the urine to a point where bacteria can no longer survive. The conclusion was that vitamin is a great way to treat urinary tract infections.[94]

Proteolytic Enzymes:

These can assist greatly for those UTI sufferers who are already taking antibiotics for their infections. The enzymes bromelain and trypsin have been shown to improve antibiotic action and clear infections faster.

In one trial, all the participants were given antibiotics to treat a urinary tract infection. Then the group was split in half. One group got tablets combining bromelain and trypsin, which were enteric-coated to protect the enzymes from stomach acid. The other group was given a placebo. *All* of the patients on enzymes had a complete recovery. Only 46% of the placebo group reported positive results.[95]

Cranberry Juice:

It may surprise you to learn that the most natural and most preferred treatment for urinary tract infections is cranberry juice. Several studies have shown that cranberry juice can be very effective in warding off UTI. The May 15, 2004 issue of *Clinical Infectious Disease* featured an article discussing these merits. It stated that cranberry juice was a great defense, especially for sexually active women who get recurring UTIs. By boosting their intake of this juice, the women saw a 50% reduction in occurrences.[96] These effects can be even more improved when combining vitamin C supplements with cranberry juice.

Vitamins vs. Drugs and Other Treatments: A Cost Comparison

Amoxil:	$25.00 or less avg. cost
Ceftin:	$100.00–$199.00 avg. cost
Cipro:	$100.00–$199.00 avg. cost
Vitamin C:	$25.00 or less avg. cost, 30-day supply
Proteolytic enzymes:	$17.00–$97.20 avg. cost, 30-day supply

Vertigo

The Condition

The terms "dizziness" and "vertigo" are often used interchangeably, but this is inaccurate, as their definitions differ. Vertigo actually creates a feeling where the world or the subject themselves seem to be whirling or tilting.

Many cases of actual vertigo are caused by a condition called benign positional paroxysmal vertigo (BPPV). It describes experiencing harmless vertigo by moving your head too fast. Vertigo can make you feel:

- Nauseous
- Fatigued
- Light-headed
- Needing to vomit
- Off balance/lack of balance

The Cause

Vertigo can result from turning your head too fast or by scenery passing by too fast, such as you might experience in a car or roller coaster. You might remember experiencing it as a child, after spinning around in circles for an extended period.

There are conditions that can bring on a bout of vertigo. These include:

- Sinusitis
- Panic attacks
- Migraine headaches

- Hypothyroidism
- High blood triglycerides
- Diabetes
- Hypoglycemia

There are drugs that can induce vertigo like ototoxic drugs and aminoglycosides. These are used by doctors in clinical settings to create vertigo in their patients.

The Cure

Here are the vitamins that will treat vertigo:

Vitamin B6:

Since the cause for vertigo can't be pinpointed, it's hard to treat. However, vitamin B6 has shown some promise, at least when treating drug-induced vertigo.

A review study looked at two double-blind trials in which B6 was used to halt drug-induced vertigo. In both studies, patients took seven doses of 40 mg daily for three days in addition to the drug. Their vertigo was far less severe than those who didn't receive the B6.[97]

This beneficial result of B6 may have to do with the vitamin's ability to build up neurotransmitters in the brain. Whereas vertigo-inducing drugs affect or block these neurotransmitters, vitamin B6 may cancel out the effects of these drugs.

Other:

If you suffer from vertigo, the herbs ginkgo and ginger can help stop nausea.

Vitamins vs. Drugs and Other Treatments: A Cost Comparison

Antivert:	$25.00–$99.00 avg. cost
Bonine:	$25.00 or less avg. cost
Dramamine II:	$25.00–$49.00 avg. cost
Vitamin B6:	$25.00 or less avg. cost, 30-day supply

Acknowledgments

The creation of any book always involves the co-operation and efforts of many individuals and *Doctors Vitamin Cures That Work* is no exception. I thank my former mentors, Dr. Kenneth Gray (University of North Carolina), Dr. Paul Munson (University of North Carolina), and Dr. Hector DeLuca (University of Wisconsin), who introduced me to the exciting world of calcium and vitamin D research. Finally, I thank my wife Shirley, and daughters Emily, Rosaline, and Karen for pitching in to allow me the time and space, let alone the use of the computer, to produce *Doctors Vitamin Cures That Work*.

Sources

1. Polidori, M.C., et al., "Plasma levels of lipophilic antioxidants in very old patients with type 2 diabetes," *Diabetes Metab Res Rev.* 2000; 16: 15–9.

2. Virtamo, J., et al., "Incidence of cancer and mortality following alpha-tocopherol and beta-carotene supplementation: a postintervention follow-up," *JAMA* July 23, 2003; 290(4): 476–485.

3. Shimon, I., et al., "Improved left ventricular function after thiamine supplementation in patients with congestive heart failure receiving long-term furosemide therapy,"*Am J Med.* 1995; 98: 485–490.

4. Schoenen, J., et al., "Effectiveness of high-dose riboflavin in migraine prophylaxis. A randomized controlled trial," *Neurology* 1998; 50: 466–470.

5. Joyce, B.J., et al., "Homocysteine Levels and the Risk of Osteoporotic Fracture," *N Engl J Med* May 13, 2004; 350: 2033–2041.

6. Tucker, K.L., et al., "Breakfast cereal fortified with folic acid, vitamin B6, and vitamin B12 increases vitamin concentrations and reduces homocysteine concentrations: a randomized trial," Am J Clin Nutr May 2004; 79(5): 805–811.

7. Baron, J.A., et al., "Folate intake, alcohol consumption, cigarette smoking, and risk of colorectal adenomas," *J Nat Can Inst.* January 7, 1998; 90: 57–62.

8. Lewis, D.P., et al., "Phenytoin-folic acid interaction," *Ann Pharmacother.* 1995; 29: 726–735.

9. Gunawardena, K., et al., "Combination therapy with vitamins C plus E inhibits surviving and human prostate cancer cell growth," *Prostate* May 15, 2004; 59(3): 319–327.

10. Peters, E.M., et al., "Vitamin C supplementation reduces the incidence of postrace symptoms of upper-respiratory-tract infection in ultramarathon runners," *Am J Clin Nutr.* February 1993; 57(2): 170–174.

11. Stewart, L.V. and Weigel, N.L., "Vitamin D and prostate cancer," *Exp Biol Med.* April 2004; 229(4): 277–284.

12. Heinonen, O.P., et al., "Prostate cancer and supplementation with alpha-tocopherol and beta-carotene: incidence and mortality in a controlled trial." *J Natl Cancer Inst.* March 18, 1998; 90(6): 440–446.

13. Feskanitch, D., et al., "Vitamin K intake and hip fractures in women: a prospective study," *Am J Clin Nutr.* 1999; 69: 74–79.

14. Wu. K., et al., "Calcium intake and risk of colon cancer in women and men," *J Natl Cancer Inst.* 2002; 94: 437–46.

15. Kaats, G.R., et al., "Effects of chromium picolinate supplementation on body composition: a randomized, double-masked, placebo-controlled study," *Curr Ther Res.* 1996; 57: 747–765.

16. Hinton, P.S., et al., "Iron supplementation improves endurance after training in iron-depleted, nonanemic women," *J Appl Physiol.* 2000; 88: 1103–1111.

17. Attias, J., et al., "Oral magnesium intake reduces permanent hearing loss induced by noise exposure," *Am J Otolaryngol.* 1994; 15: 26–32.

18. Pelkert, K., et al., "Prophylaxis of migraine with oral magnesium: results from a prospective, multi-center, placebo-controlled and double-blind randomized study," *Cephalalgia.* 1996; 16: 257–263.

19. Conlin, P.R., et al., "The effect of dietary patterns on blood pressure control in hypertensive patients: results from the Dietary Approaches to Stop Hypertension (DASH) trial," *American Journal of Hypertension* September 2000; 13(9): 949–55.

20. Ibid.

21. Hirt, M., et al., "Zinc nasal gel for the treatment of common cold symptoms: a double-blind, placebo-controlled trial," *Ear Nose Throat J.* 2000; 79: 778–781.

22. Godfrey, H.R., et al., "A randomized clinical trial on the treatment of oral herpes with topical zinc oxide/glycine," *Altern Ther Health Med.* 2001; 7: 49–54, 56.

23. Brevetti, G., et al., "European multicenter study on propionyl-L-carnitine in intermittent claudication," *J Am Coll Cardiol.* 1999; 34: 1618–1624.

24. Cacciatore, L., et al., "The therapeutic effect of L-carnitine in patients with exercise-induced stable angina: a controlled study," *Drugs Exp Clin Res.* 1991; 17: 225–235.

25. Passeri, M., et al., "Acetyl-L-carnitine in the treatment of mildly demented elderly patients," *Int J Clin Pharmacol Res.* 1990; 10: 75–79.

26. Singh, R.B., et al., "Effect of hydrosoluble coenzyme Q 10 on blood pressures and insulin resistance in hypertensive patients with coronary artery disease," *J Hum Hypertens.* 1999; 13: 203–208.

27. Reginster, J.Y., et al., "Long-term effects of glucosamine sulphate on osteoarthritis progression: a randomised, placebo-controlled clinical trial," *Lancet* 2001; 357: 251–56.

28. Richy, F., et al., "Structural and symptomatic efficacy of glucosamine and chondroitin in knee osteoarthritis: a comprehensive meta-analysis," *Arch. Int. Med.* 2003; 163: 1514–1522.

29. Griffith, R.S., et al., "Success of L-lysine therapy in frequently recurrent herpes simplex infection. Treatment and prophylaxis," *Dermatologica* 1987; 175: 183–190.

30. Baumuller, M., "The application of hydrolytic enzymes in blunt wounds to the soft tissue and distortion of the ankle joint: a double-blind clinical trial [translated from German]," *Allgemeinmedizin.* 1990; 19: 178–182.

31. Billigmann, V.P., "Enzyme therapy—an alternative in treatment of herpes zoster. A controlled study of 192 patients [translated from German]," *Fortschr Med.* 1995;

113: 43–48.

32. Shoskes, D.A., et al., "Quercetin in men with category III chronic prostatitis: a preliminary prospective, double-blind, placebo-controlled trial," *Urology* 1999; 54: 960–963.

33. Matsuyama, Y., et al., "The effect of taurine administration on patients with acute hepatitis," *Prog Clin Biol Res.* 1983; 125: 461–468.

34. Azuma, J., et al., "Double-blind randomized crossover trial of taurine in congestive heart failure," *Curr Ther Res.* 1983; 34: 543–557.

35. Meador, K., et al., "Preliminary findings of high-dose thiamine in dementia of Alzheimer's type," *J Geriatr Psychiatry Neurol* 1993; 6: 222–9; Blass, J.P., et al., "Thiamine and Alzheimer's disease. A pilot study," *Arch Neurol* 1988; 45: 833–5.

36. Sano. M., et al., "A Controlled Trial of Selegiline, Alpha-Tocopherol, or Both as Treatment for Alzheimer's Disease," *New Eng J of Med.* 1997; 336: 1216–1222.

37. Chambers, J.C., "Demonstration of rapid onset vascular endothelial dysfunction after hyperhomocysteinemia. An effect reversible with vitamin C therapy," *Circulation* March 1999; 99(9): 1156–1160.

38. Frei, B., "Ascorbic acid protects lipids in human plasma and low-density lipoprotein against oxidative damage," *Am J Clin Nutr.* 1991: 1113S–1118S.

39. Korpela, H., "Effect of selenium supplementation after acute myocardial infarction," *Res Comm Chem Pathol Pharmacol* August 1989; 65(2): 249–52.

40. Reginster, J.Y., et al., "Long-term effects of glucosamine sulphate on osteoarthritis progression: a randomised, placebo-controlled clinical trial," *Lancet* 2001; 357: 251–56.

41. Richy, F., et al., "Structural and symptomatic efficacy of glucosamine and chondroitin in knee osteoarthritis: a comprehensive meta-analysis," *Arch. Int. Med.* 2003; 163: 1514–1522.

42. Jonas, W.B., et al., "The effect of niacinamide on osteoarthritis: a pilot study," *Inflamm Res.* 1996; 45: 330–334.

43. Pattison, D.J., et al., "Vitamin C and the risk of developing inflammatory polyarthritis: prospective nested case-control study," *Annals of the Rheumatic Diseases*, 2004; 63: 843–847.

44. Collipp, P.J., et al., "Pyridoxine treatment of childhood bronchial asthma," *Ann Allergy.* 1975; 35: 93–97.

45. Zhang, S., et al., "A prospective study of folate intake and the risk of breast cancer," *JAMA* 1999; 281: 1632–7.

46. *Biophysical Research Communications* 1994; 199: 1504–8.

47. Taylor, A., et al., "Long-term intake of vitamins and carotenoids and odds of early age-related cortical and posterior subcapsular lens opacities," *Am J Clin Nutr.* 2002; 75: 540–9.

48. Jacques, P.F., et al., "Long-term vitamin C supplement use and prevalence of early age-related lens opacities," *Am J Clin Nutr.* 1997; 66(4): 911–916.

49. Taylor, A., et al., "Long-term intake of vitamins and carotenoids and odds of early age-related cortical and posterior subcapsular lens opacities," *Am J Clin Nutr.* 2002; 75: 540–9.

50. Grandjean, E.M., et al., "Efficacy of oral long-term N-acetylcysteine in chronic bronchopulmonary disease: a meta-analysis of published double-blind, placebo-controlled clinical trials," *Clin Ther.* 2000; 22: 209–221.

51. Haitt, W.R., et al., "Carnitine and acylcarnitine metabolism during exercise in humans. Dependence on skeletal muscle metabolic state," *Int J Clin Pharmacol Ther Toxicol.* 1988; 26: 269–272.

52. Griffith, R.S., et al., "Success of L-lysine therapy in frequently recurrent herpes simplex infection. Treatment and prophylaxis," *Dermatologica* 1987; 175: 183–190.

53. Godfrey, H.R., et al., "A randomized clinical trial on the treatment of oral herpes with topical zinc oxide/glycine," *Altern Ther Health Med* 2001; 7: 49–54, 56.

54. Morisco, C., et al., "Effect of coenzyme Q10 therapy in patients with congestive heart failure: A long-term multicenter randomized study," *Clin Invest.* 1993; 71(Supp 8): S134–S136.

55. Liao, F., et al., "Is low magnesium concentration a risk factor for coronary heart disease? The Atherosclerosis Risk in Communities (ARIC) Study," *Am Heart J*; 136: 480–490.

56. Woods, K.L., et al., "Intravenous magnesium sulphate in suspected acute myocardial infarction: results of the second Leicester Intravenous Magnesium Intervention Trial (LIMIT-2)," *Lancet* 1992; 339: 1553–1558.

57. Woods, K.L. and Fletcher, S., "Long-term outcome after intravenous magnesium sulphate in suspected acute myocardial infarction: the second Leicester Intravenous Magnesium Intervention Trial (LIMIT-2)," *Lancet* 1994; 343(8901): 816–819.

58. *Clin Ther* 1992; 141: 379–84.

59. Bella, R., et al., "Effect of acetyl-L-carnitine on geriatric patients suffering from dysthymic disorders," *Int J Clin Pharmaco Res.* 1990; 10: 355–360.

60. Poldinger, W., et al., "A functional-dimensional approach to depression: serotonin deficiency as a target syndrome in a comparison of 5-hydroxytryptophan and fluvoxamine," *Psychpathology* 1991; 24: 53–81.

61. Rabinovitz, H., et al., "Effect of chromium supplementation on blood glucose and lipid levels in type 2 diabetes mellitus elderly patients," *Int J Vitam Nutr Res.* 2004 May; 74(3): 178–82.

62. Bahijiri, S.M., "The effects of inorganic chromium and brewer's yeast supplementation on glucose tolerance, serum lipids and drug dosage in individuals with type 2

diabetes," *Saudi Med J* 2000; 21(9): 831–7.

63. Paolisso, G., et al., "Daily vitamin E supplements improve metabolic control but not insulin secretion in elderly type II diabetic patients," *Diabetes Care* 1993; 16(11): 1433–7.

64. Wilt, T.J., et al., "Beta-sitosterol for the treatment of benign prostatic hyperplasia: a systematic review," *BJU Int.* 1999; 83: 976–983.

65. Chen, J., et al., "Effect of oral administration of high-dose nitric oxide donor L-arginine in men with organic erectile dysfunction: results of a double blind, randomized, placebo-controlled study," *British Journal of Urology*, 1999; 83: 269–273.

66. Zorgniotti, A.W. and Lizza, E.F., "Effect of large doses of the nitric oxide precursor, L-arginine, on erectile dysfunction," *Int J Impot Res* 1994; 6: 33–6.

67. Abraham, G.E. and Flechas, J.D., "Hypothesis: Management of fibromyalgia: rationale for the use of magnesium and malic acid," *J Nutr Med* 1992; 3: 49–59.

68. Caruso, I., et al., "Double-blind study of 5-hydroxytryptophan versus placebo in the treatment of primary fibromyalgia syndrome," *J Int Med Res.* 1990; 18: 201–209.

69. Godeberge, P., "Daflon 500 mg in the treatment of hemorrhoidal disease: a demonstrated efficacy in comparison with placebo," *Angiology* 1994; 45: 574–578.

70. Singh, R.B., et al., "Effect of hydrosoluble coenzyme Q 10 on blood pressures and insulin resistance in hypertensive patients with coronary artery disease," *J Hum Hypertens.* 1999; 13: 203–208.

71. Whelton, P.K., et al., "Effects of oral potassium on blood pressure. Meta-analysis of randomized controlled clinical trials," *JAMA* 1997; 277: 1624–32.

72. Duffy, S.J., "Treatment of hypertension with ascorbic acid," *Lancet.* 1999; 354: 2048–9.

73. Boyd, S.G., et al., "Combined dietary chromium picolinate supplementation and an exercise program leads to a reduction of serum cholesterol and insulin in college-aged subjects," *J Nutr Biochem* 1998; 9: 471–5.

74. Meydani, S.N., et al., "Vitamin E supplementation and in vivo immune response in healthy elderly subjects. A randomized controlled trial," *JAMA* 1997; 277(17):1380–1386.

75. Meydani, S.N., et al., "Vitamin E and Respiratory Tract Iinfections in Elderly Nursing Home Residents: a Randomized Controlled Trial," *JAMA* August 2004; 292(7): 828–36.

76. Suhner, A., et al., "Comparative study to determine the optimal melatonin dosage form for the alleviation of jet lag," *Chronobiol Int* 1998; 15: 655–666.

77. Yang, C.M., et al., "A single dose of melatonin prevents the phase delay associated with a delayed weekend sleep pattern," *Sleep* May 2001; 24(3): 272–281.

78. Newsome, D.A., et al., "Oral zinc in macular degeneration," *Arch Ophthalmol* 1988; 106: 192–8.

79. Olson, R.J., "Supplemental dietary anoxidant vitamins and minerals in patients with macular degeneration," *J Am Coll Nutr* 1991; 10: 550.

80. Bischoff-Ferrari, H.A., et al., "Effect of Vitamin D on falls: a meta-analysis," *JAMA* 2004; 291: 1999–2006.

81. Joyce, B.A., et al., "Homocysteine Levels and the Risk of Osteoporotic Fracture," *NEJM* 2004; 350: 2033–2041.

82. Feskanich, D., et al., "Vitamin K intake and hip fractures in women: a prospective study," *Am J Clin Nutr.* 1999; 69: 74–79.

83. Combs, G.F., "Status of selenium in prostate cancer prevention," *Br J Cancer* July 2004.

84. Li, H., "A prospective study of plasma selenium levels and prostate cancer risk," *J Natl Cancer Inst.* May 2004.

85. Billigmann, V.P., "Enzyme therapy—an alternative in treatment of herpes zoster. A controlled study of 192 patients [translated from German]," *Fortschr Med.* 1995; 113: 43–48.

86. Ryan, R.E., "A double-blind clinical evaluation of bromelains in the treatment of acute sinusitis," *Headache* 1967; 7: 13–17.

87. Macknin, M.L., "Zinc lozenges for the common cold," *Cleveland Clin J Med* 1999.

88. Prasad, A.S., "Duration of symptoms and plasma cytokine levels in patients with the common cold treated with zinc acetate," *Ann Intern Med.* August 15, 2000.

89. Eby, G.A., "Reduction in duration of common colds by zinc gluconate lozenges in a double-blind study," *Antimicrob Agents Chemother* January 1984.

90. Lefebvre, P., "Jean Marquet Award. "Regeneration of the neurosensory structures in the mammalian inner ear," *Acta Otorhinolaryngol Belg.* 1997.

91 Terkelsen, L.H., "Topical application of cod liver oil ointment accelerates wound healing," *Scand J Plast Reconstr Surg Hand Surg.* March 2000.

92. Arda, H.N., "The Role of Zinc in the Treatment of Tinnitus," *Otol Neurotol* January 2003.

93. Rosenberg, S.I., "Effect of Melatonin on Tinnitus," *Laryngoscope* 1998.

94. Carlsson, S., "Effects of pH, Nitrite, and Ascorbic Acid on Nonenzymatic Nitric Oxide Generation and Bacterial Growth in Urine," *Nitric Oxide* December 2001.

95. Mori, S., et al., "The Clinical Effect of Proteolytic Enzyme Containing Bromelain and Trypsin on Urinary Tract Infection Evaluated by Double Blind Method," *Acta Obstet Gynaecol Jpn* 1972.

96. Raz, R., "Cranberry Juice and Urinary Tract Infection," *Clinical Infectious Diseases* May 2004.

97. Claussen, C.F., "Antiivertiginous Action of Vitamin B6 on Experimental Minocycline-Induced Vertigo in Man," *Arzneimittelforschung* March 1988.

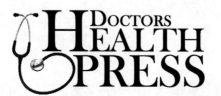